BETA-BLOCKERS IN HYPERTENSION AND ANGINA PECTORIS

BETA-BLOCKERS IN HYPERTENSION AND ANGINA PECTORIS

Different Compounds, Different Strategies

by

TON J.M. CLEOPHAS

Internist-Clinical Pharmacologist,
Department of Medicine,
Merwede Hospital Dordrecht, The Netherlands

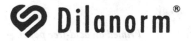

KLUWER ACADEMIC PUBLISHERS

DORDRECHT / BOSTON / LONDON

Library of Congress Cataloging-in-Publication Data

Cleophas, Ton J. M.
    Beta-blockers in hypertension and angina pectoris : different
  compounds, differenct strategies / Ton J.M. Cleophas.
      p.   cm.
    ISBN 0-7923-3516-3 (pbk. : acid-free paper)
    1. Adrenergic beta blockers.   2. Hypertension--Chemotherapy.
  3. Angina pectoris--Chemotherapy.   I. Title.
  RC684.A35C56 1995
  616.1'32'061--dc20   95-17076

ISBN 0-7923-3516-3

Published by Kluwer Academic Publishers,
P.O. Box 17, 3300 AA Dordrecht, The Netherlands.

Kluwer Academic Publishers incorporates
the publishing programmes of
D. Reidel, Martinus Nijhoff, Dr W. Junk and MTP Press.

Sold and distributed in the U.S.A. and Canada
by Kluwer Academic Publishers,
101 Philip Drive, Norwell, MA 02061, U.S.A.

In all other countries, sold and distributed
by Kluwer Academic Publishers Group,
P.O. Box 322, 3300 AH Dordrecht, The Netherlands

Printed on acid-free paper

Printed in The Netherlands

TABLE OF CONTENTS

FOREWORD

"Knowledge desires increase – it is like fire that
first must be kindled by some external agent, but
which will always afterward propagate itself".

Johnson, Letter to William Drummond August 13,
1776

The therapeutic effectiveness and safety of beta-adrenergic blocking
drugs has been well established in patients with essential hypertension
and arteriosclerotic cardiovascular disease. These drugs are useful in
primary protection against cardiovascular morbidity or mortality in
patients with essential hypertension and secondary protection (morbidity and mortality in patients with myocardial infarction). Although
there are mass action effects common to all of beta-adrenergic blocking agents, these agents differ in their effects on the RAS system,
beta blockade, norepinephrine release, CNS effects, peripheral vascular resistance, inotrophic effects, vasomotor effects, and effects on
plasma volume.

Dr. Ton J.M. Cleophas has addressed this problem of different compounds and different strategies in the use of beta-adrenergic blockers. In
Chapter 1 of this book the author deals with the problem of paradoxical
pressor responses from non cardioselective beta blockade. Chapter 2
deals with a review of the literature dealing with these pressor responses
which are usually thought to be mild and occur in situations of increased
sympathetic activity (57 references). Chapter 3 deals with the beneficial effects of alpha blockade in Raynaud's Syndrome, and the effect
of beta blockade in counteracting the alpha blocker side effects of fluid
retention and tachycardia. In Chapter 4 the author concludes that non
selective beta blockers largely diminish the orthostatic hypotension in
diabetes with hyperadrenergic postural hypotension and vagal neuropathy. The author reports on studies in Chapter 5 of a pressor effect of non
cardioselective beta blockers in mildly hypertensive patients acutely

hospitalized. In Chapter 6 a randomized study is presented demonstrating that in spite of equipotent doses, metropolol causes a larger reduction of blood pressure than propranolol. Chapter 7 compares the effects of celiprolol and propranolol in unstable angina pectoris. The 8th and final Chapter involved additional discussion on paradoxical pressor effects of non selective beta blockers, originally discussed in Chapter 1. Dr. Cleophas's book based chiefly on observations and studies addresses a subject that has been neglected in the literature.

Robert B. Kaïmansohn, M.D.
President-Elect, American College of Angiology
F.A.C.P., F.C.C.P., F.A.C.A., F.A.C.C., F.I.C.A.
Clinical Professor of Medicine (Cardiology),
UCLA Medical Center, Los Angeles, California
Attending Physician in Cardiology, Cedars Sinai
Medical Center, Los Angeles, California

PREFACE

Because of their excellent record of efficacy and safety, beta-blockers have become one of the commonly prescribed classes of drugs to be used in the treatment of hypertension and angina pectoris, and for the prevention of myocardial infarction. In situations of increased sympathetic activity, however, a pressor effect interferes with their otherwise beneficial effects on blood pressure and myocardial oxygen demand. The present work reviews the literature on this subject so far. The pressor effect, although a reproducible phenomenon of nonselective beta-blockers, is rarely seen with selective beta-blockers. Although the clinical relevance of the phenomenon in terms of permanent harm has not been elucidated so far, we may ask do we require the very proof of it by exposing mankind to a less effective compound and isn't it time to replace nonselective by selective beta-blockers more systematically.

ACKNOWLEDGEMENTS

This work reports studies that have been performed at the outpatient clinic (Head Dr. J.F.M. Fennis) of the Department of Medicine (Head Prof. Dr. A. van 't Laar) of the St. Radboudhospital, Nijmegen and Department of Medicine, Merwede Hospital, Sliedrecht, The Netherlands. I wish to thank all the members of these departments who have assisted in the completion of this work, particularly Dr. Kauw. I am also very grateful to Mr. H.J.J. van Lier and Dr. K. Zwinderman, Statistical Consultants for their statistical analyses. I wish to thank the nurses of the outpatient clinic (Head Mrs. T.C.M. de Klerk and Mrs. T.T.M. Hoogenbosch) for their assistance and readiness to serve as testperson. The randomisation of patients and preparations of therapies were performed by Mrs. Drs. J.C.L. Benneker of the Department of Pharmacy. The figures were designed by Mr. C.P. Nicolasen and Mr. A. Jannink. Photographical reproductions were made at the Departments of Medical Photography (Mr. A.Th.A. Reijnen and Mr. A. Jannink). The literature was collected at the Medical Department of the University Library (Head Mr. E. de Graaff). Furthermore, thanks to Mrs. Babette Gladpootjes for carefully typing manuscripts. Celiprolol was kindly provided by Rhone Poulenc Rorer B.V., The Netherlands.

Ton J.M. Cleophas

CHAPTER 1

INTRODUCTION AND OUTLINE OF CURRENT WORK

1.1. Introduction

Although many more mechanisms are involved in the modulation of vascular tone as well as blood pressure, the balance between vasoconstrictive alpha-receptors and vasodilatory beta-receptors is considered to be one of them. The neurotransmitter norepinephrine, when released from sympathetic nerve endings, will normally stimulate both vasoconstrictive alpha-receptors and vasodilatory beta-receptors (Figure 1), and the net effect will be little change in vascular tone or level of blood pressure. However, when postsynaptic alpha-receptors have been blocked beforehand by the alpha-blocker phenoxybenzamine, then sympathetic nerve stimulation is likely to cause a vasodilator (beta-receptor) action. Similarly, when postsynaptic beta-receptors have been blocked by the nonselective beta-blocker propranolol, sympathetic nerve stimulation will cause a vasoconstrictor (alpha-receptor) action. These very effects can be simulated by intravenous administration of small doses of epinephrine in patients pretreated with either an alpha- or a beta-blocker. Figure 2 shows a sharp depressor effect of epinephrine after pretreatment with 10 mg of phenoxybenzamine intravenously, and, in addition, a sharp pressor effect of epinephrine after pretreatment with 10 mg of propranolol intravenously. Studies on alpha- or beta-blockers in patients with hypertension or angina pectoris did not routinely account for underlying levels of sympathetic activity. Probably this is why paradoxical pressor effects of beta-blockers have not been generally recognized and also why alpha-blockers have been classified as generally weak hypotensive agents. In this booklet an overview will be presented of studies focusing on situations of increased sympathetic activity. The pressor effect of nonselective beta-blockers appears to be a highly reproducible phenomenon. Although there are no reports of persistent harm being done by this phenomenon, it does make sense to choose instead of a nonselective, a selective beta-blocker which large-

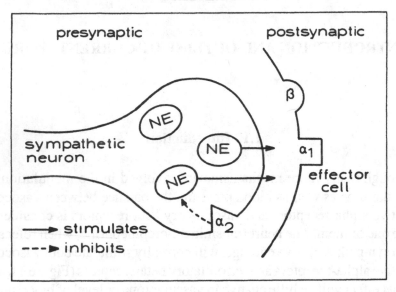

Fig. 1.   Schematic representation of sympathetic nerve ending on a blood vessel and of some of the adrenergic receptors. NE = norepinephrine.

ly lacks this phenomenon and is equally effective for the treatment of patients with hypertension and angina pectoris.

1.2. Outline of Current Work

Paradoxical pressor responses from noncardioselective beta-blockers have been published in more than sixty scientific papers in international medical journals. The pressor responses are probably due to alpha-receptor-mediated vasoconstriction unopposed by beta-2-receptor-mediated vasodilation. In situations of increased sympathetic activity this mechanism may override the otherwise hypotensive properties of the noncardioselective beta-blockers. Some patients seem to be at risk; e.g., patients with unstable diabetes type I, sportsmen who perform a lot of isometric exercise, and perhaps also heavy smokers (Chapter 2). In them the preference for a cardioselective beta-blocker has been recommended by my group. The pressor effect was beneficial in patients on alpha-blockers (Chapter 3) and in patients with orthostatic hypotension (Chapter 4). In 1988, we reviewed the articles on this subject published at that time. Our conclusions have been adopted by Goodman and Gilman, *The Pharmacological Basis of Therapeutics*

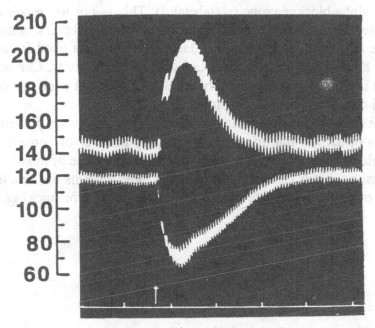

Fig. 2. Responses of blood pressure to 0.2 mg of epinephrine intravenously (arrow) after pretreatment with either 10 mg of the alpha-blocker phenoxybenzamine intravenously (lower record) or 10 mg of propranolol intravenously (upper record). After blockade of vasodilatory beta-receptors epinephrine exerts a pressor effect due to stimulation of vasoconstrictive alpha-receptors. After blockade of the vasoconstrictive alpha-receptors, it exerts a depressor action due to stimulation of vasodilatory beta-receptors.

(New York, Pergamon Press, 1991). In recent controlled and double-blind studies the pressor effect has been demonstrated during increased sympathetic activity due to acute hospitalization (Chapter 5), surgery (Chapter 6), and unstable angina pectoris (Chapter 7). Although the clinical relevance of the phenomenon in terms of permanent harm has not been elucidated so far, we may ask: do we require the very proof of it by exposing mankind to a less effective and potentially hazardous compound? Beta-2-blockade, if not hazardous, does not seem to reduce blood pressure either, although initially it was thought to do so (Chapter 8). We should add that there are more reasons for choosing a beta-1-selective blocker, e.g., bronchus constriction especially in patients with chronic obstructive pulmonary disease, delayed recovery from hypoglycemia in diabetes mellitus, and severe hypertriglyceridemia. The pressor effects have also been described with nonselective beta-blockers with intrinsic sympathicomimetic activity (ISA) or with additional alpha-blocker property (labetalol). This is not too much of a surprise because these compounds do block beta-2-receptors, although maybe less vigorously. Moreover, labetalol is not that good for additional alpha-1-blockade since it lacks alpha-1-selectivity. Carvedilol which is alpha-1-selective may be a better choice, but even this compound does block beta-2-receptors.

The reverse of the medal is that the results of secondary prevention studies of myocardial infarction are slightly in favor of nonselective beta-blockers. Maybe, this is partly due to the presence of mostly normotensives in this category. Still, even in these patients the beneficial effect of nonselective beta-blockade is lost by the factor smoking.

CHAPTER 2

PRESSOR RESPONSES FROM NONCARDIOSELECTIVE
BETA-BLOCKERS

This chapter reviews more than fifty papers dealing with pressor responses from noncardioselective beta-blockers. It is concluded that the responses are usually mild. They occur mainly in situations of increased sympathetic activity. Therefore some patients seem to be at risk, e.g., patients with unstable diabetes type 1, sportsmen performing isometric exercise, and heavy smokers. In orthostatic hypotension, noncardioselective beta-blockers may be beneficial. Cardiac output tends, however, to decrease, and patients with orthostatic hypotension will probably not benefit from this effect.

2.1. Introduction

About 60% of the beta-blockers are prescribed for the treatment of hypertension. In Europe 35% of hypertensive patients receive beta-blockers, and in the United States about 25% [1]. Despite their popularity it is known that their hypotensive activity is sometimes slight or even absent, e.g., in low renin states [2]. Pressor responses have even been described, especially with the so-called noncardioselective beta-blockers. The present study analyzes the published data in light of the following questions:
1. When do these pressor responses occur?
2. Are they substantial or just slight and unimportant?
3. Are there patients at risk for these pressor responses?
4. Can they be beneficial, e.g., in situations of hypotension?

2.2. The First Reports

More than ten years ago the first reports on pressor responses from noncardioselective beta-blockers were published. Tarazi [3] and Blum

[4] reported unexpected pressor effects from propranolol in situations of emotional stress. Similar data were observed by Drayer [5], studying low renin hypertension with increased sympathetic activity. Finally the effect was observed in patients with untreated pheochromocytoma [6, 7]. The most consistent finding in all these studies was a situation of increased sympathetic activity. It was hypothesized that alpha-receptor-mediated vasoconstriction unopposed by beta-2-receptor-mediated vasodilation might be responsible. In situations of increased sympathetic activity this mechanism might override the otherwise hypotensive activities of noncardioselective beta-blockers. Pursuing this hypothesis, a number of investigators then started to design controlled trials to provide more evidence on this subject and to compare cardioselective and noncardioselective blockers in these conditions. These studies are discussed next.

2.3. Controlled Studies Designed to Demonstrate Pressor Responses from Noncardioselective Beta-Blockers

INFUSIONS OF EPINEPHRINE

Figure 1, displaying the data of van Herwaarden [8] shows what happens if epinephrine is administered to hypertensive patients who have been receiving beta-blockers for a period of time. In the group taking metoprolol – the cardioselective group – blood pressure hardly changes. In the propranolol group – the noncardioselective group – there is a substantial rise of mean blood pressure. The placebo effect on systolic pressure was ascribed to increase of cardiac output after epinephrine, since heart rate rises after placebo but not after beta-blockade. This study strongly supports the conclusion that noncardioselective beta-blockers can indeed cause unexpected pressor responses. By now this finding has been reported by three more papers [9–11], so the effect can not be easily ignored. Daily life stress involves, however, more complicated processes than the infusion of epinephrine does.

PHARMACOLOGIC STRESS

Figure 2, displaying the study of Trap-Jensen [12], shows the effect of nicotine during administration of saline, propranolol, or the car-

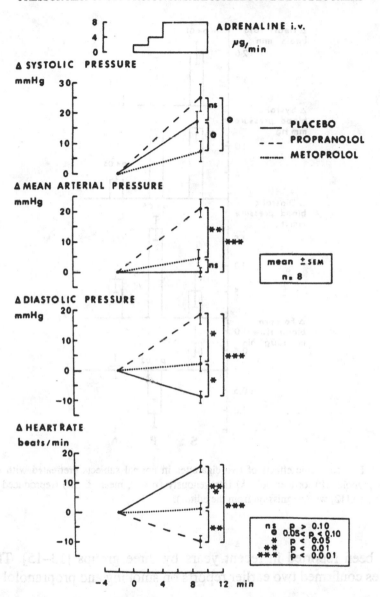

Fig. 1.   Influence of infusion of epinephrine on blood pressure and heart rate in hypertensive subjects pretreated for four weeks with placebo or different beta-blockers (reproduced from van Herwaarden [8] with permission from the editor).

dioselective beta-blocker atenolol. Propranolol caused a marked rise in diastolic pressure and peripheral resistance. The effect of atenolol was slight and insignificant. The same effects after chronic beta-blockade

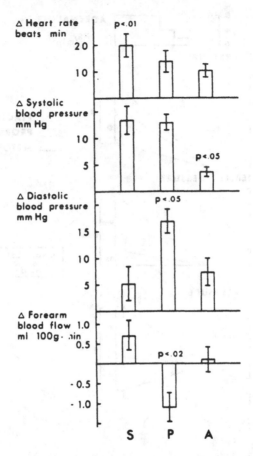

Fig. 2. Hemodynamic effects of two cigarettes in normal subjects pretreated with saline (S), propranolol (P), or atenolol (A) intravenously ($n = 7$, mean $\pm$ SE) (reproduced from Trap-Jensen [12] with permission from the editor).

have been reported in recent years by three groups [13–15]. These studies confirmed two earlier reports on smoking and propranolol [16, 17].

Nicotine is just like caffeine and insulin – a drug in daily life that causes a substantial rise of plasma epinephrine [18–20]. It can be used as a model for pharmacologic stress. Moreover, insulin has been quite successful in demonstrating pressor responses from noncardioselective beta-blockers. The first reports were from Lloyd-Mostyn [21] and from Davidson [22] a decade ago. Figure 3 shows a plot of data of Lloyd-Mostyn. After administration of insulin, blood pressure goes down.

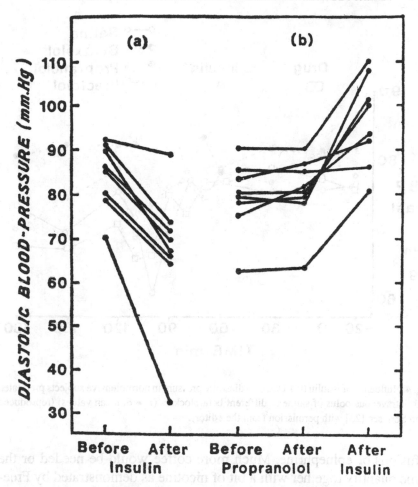

Fig. 3. Influence of insulin (0.2 U/kg) on diastolic pressure in normal subjects with or without prior intravenous administration of propranolol (10 mg) (reproduced from Lloyd-Mostyn [21] with permission from the author and editor).

However, after pretreatment with propranolol, blood pressure goes up. During this decade, seven more reports [23–29] have appeared confirming these results, for example, the study of Sonksen [23] (Figure 4) and the study of Lauridsen [25] (Figure 5).

What about caffeine? It has been less successful than nicotine and insulin. Smits [30], for example, could not demonstrate a difference between cardioselective and noncardioselective beta-blockers. He ascribed this failure to an increase of plasma epinephrine of less than 200%, which was the lowest level to cause a pressor response to

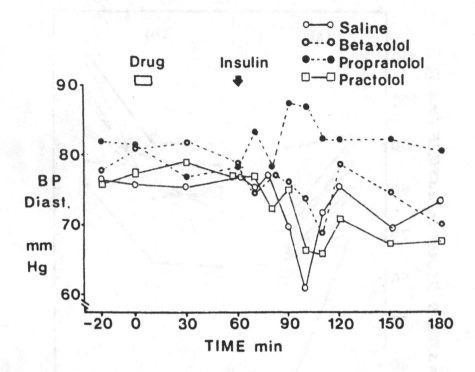

Fig. 4. Influence of insulin (0.1 U/kg) on diastolic pressure in normotensive subjects pretreated with intravenous bolus of saline or different beta-blockers ($n = 6$, mean values) (reproduced from Sonksen [23] with permission from the editor).

infusions of epinephrine. Much more coffee would be needed or the same quantity together with a bit of nicotine as demonstrated by Freestone [31] (Table I). The noncardioselective beta-blockers caused a firm increase of blood pressure. The selective beta-blocker atenolol had only a small and insignificant effect. The placebo-effect was connected with increase of cardiac output, presumably absent after beta-blockers.

OTHER TYPES OF STRESS

Other types of stress used to study differences between the two beta-blockers are environmental stress, such as cold, loud noise, pain; mental stress, such as arithmetic; physical stress, such as handgrip and different types of dynamic exercise. Most of these stress models cause smaller increases of catecholamines in the laboratory than the infusion of catecholamines does [32]. Nonetheless, subtle differences between

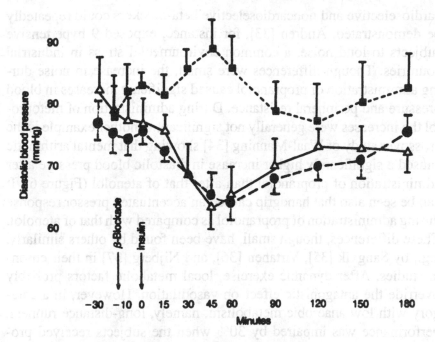

Fig. 5. Influence of insuline (0.2 U/kg) on diastolic pressure in normal subjects ($n = 12$, mean ± SE) pretreated with intravenous bolus of saline (△), atenolol (•), and propranolol (■) (reproduced from Lauridsen [25] with permission from the editor).

TABLE I

Influence of 500 ml coffee plus 2 cigarettes in hypertensive habitual smokers pretreated for 6 weeks with placebo or different beta-blockers ($n = 8$, mean values). (Reproduced from Freestone [31] with permission from the editor).

	Systolic BP (mm Hg)	Diastolic BP (mm Hg)	Pulse Rate (beats/min)
Propranolol	8.5*	8.0***	5.8*
Oxprenolol	12.1**	9.1**	4.7*
Atenolol	5.2	4.4	5.3***
Placebo	9.8**	8.5***	11.1**

* $p < 0.05$ vs baseline values.

** $p < 0.01$ vs baseline values.

*** $p < 0.001$ vs baseline values.

cardioselective and noncardioselective beta-blockers could repeatedly be demonstrated. Andren [33], for instance, exposed 9 hypertensive subjects to loud noise, a common environmental stress in industrial countries. Though differences were small, the increase in noise during administration of propranolol caused significant increases in blood pressure and peripheral resistance. During administration of metoprolol the increases were generally not significant. Another example is the crossover study of Waal-Manning [34] showing that mental arithmetic caused a significantly higher increase in diastolic blood pressure after administration of propranolol than after that of atenolol (Figure 6). It can be seen also that handgrip caused an accentuated pressor response during administration of propranolol as compared with that of atenolol. These differences, though small, have been found by others similarly, e.g., by Sangvik [35], Virtanen [36], and Nijberg [37] in their chronic studies. After dynamic exercise, local metabolic factors probably override the antagonistic effect on vasodilation. However, in a category with low anaerobic metabolism, namely, long-distance runners, performance was impaired by 30% when the subjects received propranolol but by only 10% when they received atenolol. Karlson [38] attributed this effect to prevention of beta-2-receptor-mediated vasodilation. Blood pressures were not registered in this study.

Atsmon [39] did register blood pressures when he administered propranolol or placebo to patients with acute psychosis; 67% had increased urine levels of catecholamines. In most of them and in 50% of the whole group, hypertension (defined as a diastolic pressure above 100 mm Hg) developed after administration of propranolol and disappeared after discontinuation of the drug.

2.4. Other Studies Demonstrating Pressor Responses from Noncardioselective Beta-Blockers

ALPHA-BLOCKADE

As can be seen, the pressor responses appear exclusively in situations of increased sympathetic activity. An increased release of norepinephrine from sympathetic nerve terminals and increased levels of plasma norepinephrine are consistent findings in patients on alpha-blockers. Consequently, this may be a situation to demonstrate a pressor response

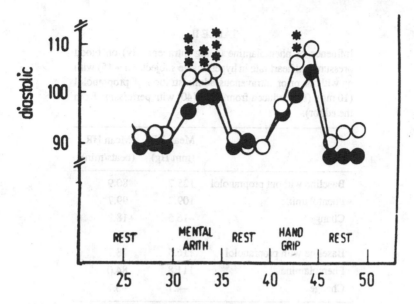

Fig. 6.   Influence of mental arithmetic and handgrip on diastolic pressure in hypertensive patients ($n = 27$, mean) pretreated for eight weeks with atenolol (•) or nonselective beta-blockers (○), (equipotent doses of exprenolol, pindolol, or propranolol) (reproduced from Waal-Manning [34] with permission from the editor). ** $p < 0.03$ atenolol vs nonselective blockers; *** $p < 0.01$ atenolol vs nonselective blockers.

from beta-blockers as well. Table II shows the data of Zahir [40]. In young hypertensive patients the nonselective alpha-blocker phentolamine caused a mean fall in blood pressure of 16.5 mm Hg and an increase in mean heart rate of 19 beats/min. After pretreatment with propranolol the mean fall in blood pressure was only 4.7 mm Hg, and heart rate hardly increased. Propranolol apparently antagonizes not only the increase in heart rate but also the hypotensive activity of alpha-blockers.

Some authors have found that alpha-blocker-induced orthostatic hypotension can be prevented by the addition of a beta-blocker to the alpha-blocker [41–43]. This may be due to a mechanism similar to our finding. We have had the opportunity to study the effect of noncardioselective beta-blockade in alpha-blocked Raynaud-patients [44, 45]. After they received 20 mg phenoxybenzamine for eight weeks, we saw no decrease in blood pressure but much fluid retention, which is known to antagonize the hypotensive activity of alpha-blockers. After the addition of the noncardioselective beta-blocker sotalol for eight weeks, we

TABLE II

Influence of phentolamine (5 mg intravenously) on blood pressure and heart rate in hypertensive subjects ($n = 15$) with or without prior intravenous administration of propranolol (10 mg). (Reproduced from Zahir [40] with permission from the editor).

	Mean BP (mm Hg)	Mean HR (beats/min)
Baseline without propranolol	125.7	80.9
Phentolamine	109.2	99.7
Change	–16.5	+18.8
Baseline with propranolol	116.5	78.7
Phentolamine	111.8	84.0
Change	–4.7*	+6.7*

* $p < 0.01$ with vs without propranolol.

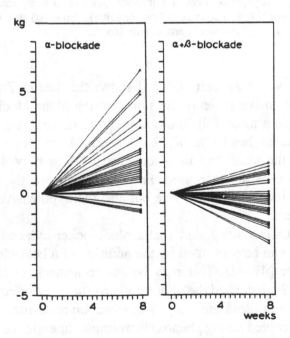

Fig. 7.   Influence of alpha-blockade (phenoxybenzamine 20 mg daily) or alpha- plus beta-blockade (phenoxybenzamine 20 mg and sotalol 80 mg daily) on fluid retention in patients with Raynaud's syndrome.

also saw no decrease in blood pressure, but fluid retention was prevented completely (Figure 7). A pressor response antagonizing the hypotensive alpha-blocker effect and thus antagonizing fluid retention seemed a plausible explanation. Orthostatic and exercise hypotension were also not seen during our experiments.

AUTONOMIC NEUROPATHY

Other forms of orthostatic hypotension have also been treated successfully with beta-blockers, as reported in about ten papers [46–55], mostly case reports. To eliminate potential biases as seen with uncontrolled studies, we recently performed a double-blind, placebo-controlled study in 11 patients with symptoms of orthostatic hypotension [56]. All patients had vagal neuropathy and largely elevated levels of plasma catecholamines as seen with hyperadrenergic diabetic syndrome. Supine and standing values were compared after administration of placebo and of different beta-agonists and beta-antagonists (Figure 8). After placebo, standing caused a significant fall in blood pressure. The beta-2 agonist terbutaline (5 mg) and the beta-1 + 2 agonist orciprenaline (10 mg) did not reduce the fall in systolic pressure on standing. The beta-1 blocker with intrinsic sympathicomimetic activity (ISA) acebutolol (200 mg) and the beta-1 blocker without ISA metoprolol (50 mg) did not reduce the fall either. Only the noncardioselective blockers propranolol (40 mg) and pindolol (5 mg) significantly reduced or practically abolished the fall. The effect in a three-week trial with pindolol (15 mg/day) was similar. As cardiac output was reduced, the effect was ascribed, not to positive inotropic ISA effect, but to prevention of beta-2 receptor vasodilation.

2.5. Conclusions

Reports of pressor responses from noncardioselective beta-blockers have been published in more than fifty scientific papers in leading medical journals. Because of these reports, should we prefer a cardioselective to a noncardioselective beta-blocker to treat our patients with hypertension and angina pectoris? Note that the pressor responses are usually mild. The increase in mean blood pressure in the controlled studies has never been more than 30 mm Hg and is mostly

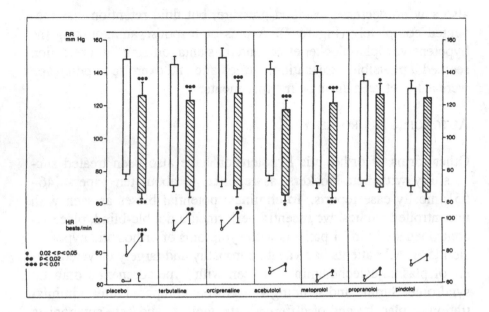

Fig. 8. Comparisons of supine and standing blood pressures and heart rates on placebo and medications (mean ± SE) in diabetics with symptoms of postural hypotension ($n = 11$). Probabilities relate to the difference between supine and standing values. Reproduced from Cleophas [56].

around 10 mm Hg. If we discontinue the noncardioselective beta-blockers, then we discontinue the theoretical advantage of presynaptic beta-2-blockade, which has been considered one of the hypotensive mechanisms of noncardioselective beta-blockers [57]. The pressor responses are probably due to alpha-receptor-mediated vasoconstriction unopposed by beta-2-receptor-mediated vasodilation. In situations of increased sympathetic activity this mechanism may override the otherwise hypotensive properties of the noncardioselective beta-blockers. Therefore, some patients seem to be at risk; e.g., patients with unstable diabetes type 1, sportsmen who perform a lot of isometric exercise, and perhaps also heavy smokers. In them the preference for a cardioselective beta-blocker might be reasonable. In the other patients studied till now data are limited. Not yet studied have been stress situations such as surgery, angina pectoris, and myocardial infarction. The problem seems certainly important enough to initiate further studies on this subject. In orthostatic hypotension noncardioselective beta-blockers may be beneficial. Cardiac output tends, however, to decrease, and patients with orthostatic hypotension will probably not benefit from this effect. Moreover, sympathetic activity in these patients is frequently low. In our opinion, therefore, this indication calls for caution.

Acknowledgements

I am indebted to Westminster Publications INC, New York, NY, for kindly granting permission to use part of a paper previously published in ANGIOLOGY (1988; 39: 587–596).

References

1. Helfland WH: A market analyst's perspective on hypertension and its treatment. In: Hypertension and the Angiotensin System: Therapeutic Approaches, ed. by Doyle AE, Bearn AG. New York: Raven Press, 1984, pp 20–24.
2. Laragh JH: Conceptual diagnostic and therapeutic dimensions of the renin system. In: Hypertension and the Angiotensin System: Therapeutic Approaches, ed. by Doyle AE, Bearn AG. New York: Raven Press, 1984, p 67.
3. Tarazi RC, Dustan HP: Beta-adrenergic blockade in hypertension. Practical and theoretical implications of long-term hemodynamic variations. Am J Cardiol 29: 633–640, 1972.
4. Blum J, Atsmon A, Steiner M, et al.: Paradoxical rise in blood pressure during propranolol treatment. Br Med J 2: 623, 1975.
5. Drayer JIM, Keim HJ, Weber MA, et al.: Unexpected pressor response to propranolol in essential hypertension on interaction between renin, aldosterone, and sympathetic activity. Am J Med 60: 897–903, 1976.
6. Nickerson M, Collier B: Beta-adrenergic blocking agents. In: The Pharmacological Basis of Therapeutics, ed. by Goodman LS and Gilman A. New York: MacMillan, 1975, pp 547–552.
7. Bravo EL, Gifford RW: Pheochromocytoma: Diagnosis, localization and management. N Engl J Med 311: 1298–1303, 1987.
8. van Herwaarden CLA: Selective and non-selective beta-blockade in hypertension. Thesis, 1978, Nijmegen, The Netherlands.
9. Johnson G: Influence of metoprolol and propranolol on haemodynamic effects induced by adrenaline and physical work. Acta Pharmacol Toxicol 36s: 59–68, 1975.
10. Houben H, Thien T, deBoo T, et al.: Influence of selective and nonselective beta-adrenoceptor blockade on the haemodynamic effect of adrenaline during combined antihypertensive drug therapy. Clin Sci 57s: 387–389, 1979.
11. Houben H, Thien T, van 't Laar A: Effect of low-dose epinephrine infusion on haemodynamics after selective and nonselective beta-blockade in hypertension. Clin Pharmacol Ther 31: 685–690, 1982.
12. Trap-Jensen J, Carlsen JE, Svendsen TL, et al.: Cardiovascular and adrenergic effects of cigarette smoking during immediate nonselective and selective beta adrenergic blockade in humans. Eur J Clin Invest 9: 181–183, 1979.

13. Ramsay LE, Freestone S: Effects of chronic beta-blockade on the pressor response to cigarette smoking. Br J Clin Pharmacol 15: 596–597, 1983.

14. Cuspidi S, Aliprandi PL, Cavalline F: Effects of short- and long-term beta-blockade on changes in blood pressure caused by cigarette smoking in normotensive and hypertensive subjects. Drugs 25s2: 148–149, 1983.

15. Fogari J, Parini A, Finardi G: Cardiovascular response to cigarette smoking during adrenergic block in essential hypertension. Drugs 25s2: 149–150, 1983.

16. Brandsborg O, Christensen NJ, Galbo H, et al.: The effect of exercise, smoking, and propranolol on serum gastrin in patients with duodenal ulcer and in vagotomized subjects. Scand J Clin Lab Invest 38: 441–446, 1978.

17. Westfall TC, Cipolloni PB, Edmundowicz AC: Influence of propranolol on haemodynamic changes and plasma catecholamine levels following cigarette smoking and nicotine. Proc Soc Exp Biol Med 123: 174–179, 1966.

18. Robertson RP, Porte D: Adrenergic modulation of basal insulin secretion in man. Diabetes 22: 1–8, 1973.

19. Cryer PE, Haymond MW, Santiago JV, et al.: Norepinephrine and epinephrine release and adrenergic mediation of smoking-associated haemodynamic and metabolic events. N Engl J Med 295: 573–577, 1976.

20. Houben H: Haemodynamic effects of stress during selective and nonselective beta-blockade. Thesis, 1982, Nijmegen, The Netherlands.

21. Lloyd-Mostyn RH, Oram S: Modification by propranolol of cardiovascular effects on induced hypoglycemia. Lancet 1: 1312–1315, 1979.

22. Davidson N, Corrall RJ, Shaw TR, et al.: Observations in man of hypoglycemia during selective and nonselective beta-blockade. Scott Med J 22; 69–72, 1976.

23. Sonksen PH, Brown PM, Saunders J: Metabolic effects of betaxolol during hypoglycemia and exercise in normal volunteers. In: L.E.R.S., Vol 1, ed. by Morselli PL, et al. New York: Raven Press, 1983, pp 143–155.

24. Ostmann J, Aner J, Haglund K, et al.: Effect of metoprolol and alprenolol on the metabolic, hormonal, and haemodynamic responses to insulin-induced hypoglycemia in hypertensive insulin-dependent diabetics. Acta Med Scand 211: 381–385, 1982.

25. Lauridsen UB, Christensen MJ, Lyngsoe J: Effects of nonselective and beta-1 selective blockade on glucose metabolism and hormonal response during insulin-induced hypoglycaemia in normal man. J Clin Endocrinol Metab 56: 876–882, 1983.

26. Kolendorf J, Aerenlund Jensen H, Holst JJ, et al.: Effects of acute selective beta-adrenergic blockade on hormonal and cardiovascular response to insulin-induced hypoglycemia in insulin-dependent diabetic patients. Scand J Clin Lab Invest 42: 69–74, 1982.

27. Pape J: Blood pressure and pulse response to insulin during nonselective and selective beta-blockade. Acta Med Scand 210s1: 105–108, 1981.

28. Nilsson OR, Karlberg BE, Soderberg A: Plasma catecholamines and cardiovascular responses to hypoglycemia in hyperthyroidism before and during treatment with metoprolol and propranolol. J Clin Endocrinol Metab 50: 906–911, 1980.

29. Ryan JR, Lacorte W, Jain A, et al.: Response of diabetics treated with atenolol or propranolol to insulin-induced hypoglycemia. Drugs 25s2: 256–257, 1983.

30. Smits P: Coffee and blood pressure, a pharmacological study on the circulatory effects of coffee and caffeine. Thesis, 1986, Nijmegen, The Netherlands.

31. Freestone S, Ramsay LE: Effect of beta-blockade on the pressor response to coffee plus smoking in patients with mild hypertension. Drugs 25s: 141–145, 1983.

32. Robertson D, Jonson GA, Robertson RM, et al.: Comparative assessment of stimuli that release neuronal and adrenomedullary catecholamines in man. Circulation 59: 637–643, 1979.

33. Andren L, Hansson L, Bjorkman M: Haemodynamic effects of noise exposure before and after beta-1 selective and nonselective beta-adrenoceptor blockade in patients with essential hypertension. Clin Sci 61s: 89–91, 1981.

34. Waal-Manning HJ: Atenolol and three nonselective beta-blockers in hypertension. Clin Pharmacol Ther 25: 8–18, 1979.

35. Sangvik K, Stokkeland M, Lindseth EM, et al.: Circulation reaction at rest and during isometric exercise in hypertension patients: Influence of different adrenergic beta-adrenoceptor antagonists. Pharmatherapeutica 1: 71–83, 1976.

36. Virtanen K, Janne J, Frick MH: Response of blood pressure and plasma norepinephrine to propranolol, metoprolol and clonidine during isometric exercise and dynamic exercise in hypertensive patients. Eur J Clin Pharmacol 21: 275–279, 1982.

37. Nijberg G: Blood pressure and heart rate during sustained handgrip in hypertensive patients taking placebo, a non-selective beta-blocker and a selective beta-blocker. Curr Ther Res 22: 828–838, 1977.

38. Karlson J: Muscle fiber composition, short-term beta-1 and beta-2 blockade and endurance exercise performance in healthy young men. Drugs 25s: 241–246, 1983.

39. Atsmon A, Blum I, Steiner M, et al.: Further studies with propranolol in psychotic patients: Relation to initial psychiatric state, urinary catecholamines, and 3-methoxy-4-hydroxyglycol excretion. Psychopharmacologia 27: 249–254, 1972.

40. Zahir M, Gould L: Phentolamine and beta-adrenergic receptors. J Clin Pharmacol 11: 197–203, 1971.

41. Kinceaid-Smith P: Prazosin in the treatment of hypertension. Med J Aust s2: 27–28, 1977.

42. Majid PA, Meeran MK, Sharma B, et al.: Alpha- and beta-adrenergic receptor blockade in the treatment of hypertension. Br Heart J 36: 588–596, 1974.

43. Johnson BJ, Labrooy J, Munro-Faure AD: The antihypertensive efficacy of combined alpha- and beta-adrenoceptor blockade with phentolamine-oxprenolol or labetalol. Clin Sci 51s: 505–507, 1976.

44. Cleophas TJM: Adrenergic receptor agonists and antagonists in Raynaud's syndrome. Thesis, 1982, Nijmegen, The Netherlands.

45. Cleophas TJM, Fennis JFM, van 't Laar A: Alpha- and beta-blockade and beta-stimulation in Raynaud's syndrome: A double-blind, placebo-controlled, single-dose study. Angiology 36: 219–225, 1985.

46. Streeten DH, Kerr CB, Prior JC, et al.: Hyperbradikinism: A new orthostatic syndrome. Lancet 11: 1048–1053, 1972.

47. Miller AJ, Cohen HC, Glick G: Propranolol in the treatment of orthostatic tachycardia associated with orthotatic hypotension. Am Heart J 88: 493–495, 1974.

48. Chobanian AV, Volicer L, Liang CS, et al.: Use of propranolol in the treatment of idiopathic orthostatic hypotension. Trans Assoc Am Physicians 90: 324–334, 1977.

49. Brevetti G, Chiarello M, Lavecchia G, et al.: Effect of propranolol in a case of orthostatic hypotension. Br Heart J 41: 245–248, 1979.

50. Frewinn DB, Leonello PP, Benhall PK, et al.: Pindolol in orthostatic hypotension. Possible therapy? Med J Aust 1: 128, 1980.

51. Robson D: Pindolol in postural hypotension. Lancet 11: 1280, 1981.

52. Man in 't Veld AJ, Schalekamp MADH: Pindolol acts as beta-adrenoceptor agonist in orthostatic hypotension: Therapeutic implications. Br Med J 282: 929–931, 1981.

53. Man in 't Veld AJ, Boomsma F, Schalekamp MADH: Effects of beta-adrenoceptor agonists and antagonists in patients with peripheral autonomic neuropathy. Br J Clin Pharmacol 13s: 367–374, 1982.
54. Boesen F, Andersen EB, Kanstrup Hansen JL, et al.: Behandling af invaliderende ortostatik hypotension med pindolol ved diabetish autonom neuropati. Vidensk Praksis (August), pp 2335–2338, 1982.
55. Bijl CH, Cleophas TJM, Kauw FHW: Pindolol in orthostatic hypotension. Angiology 36: 684, 1985.
56. Cleophas TJM, Kauw FHW, Bijl CH, et al.: Effects of beta-adrenergic receptor agonists and antagonists in diabetics with symptoms of postural hypotension: A double-blind placebo-controlled study. Angiology 37: 855–862, 1986.
57. Langer SZ: Presynaptic receptors and their role in the regulation of transmitter release. Br J Pharmacol 60: 481–497, 1977.

CHAPTER 3

ALPHA-BLOCKER INDUCED HYPOTENSION AND FLUID RETENTION PREVENTED BY NONSELECTIVE BETA-BLOCKERS

In a double-blind placebo controlled crossover trial of 24 weeks 31 patients with Raynaud's syndrome were treated with the alpha-blocker phenoxybenzamine (10–20 mg daily) and with the combination of the alpha-blocker phenoxybenzamine (10–20 mg daily) and the beta-blocker sotalol (40–80 mg daily). A favorable effect on recovery of finger temperature after finger cooling was demonstrated after alpha-blockade as compared to the before treatment situation. This favorable effect was not different when the group received the combined alpha- and beta-blockade. The blood pressure was not influenced by either of the 2 medications. Fluid retention appeared with alpha-blockade and was absent with combined alpha- and beta-blockade. Decrease of heart rate occurred with alpha-plus beta-blockade and was absent with alpha-blockade alone. Clinical symptoms of Raynaud's syndrome were equally alleviated by the two medications. Common, and equally frequent side effects of the two medications were nasal congestion, disturbed ejaculation and potence, dry mouth, exercise-induced, and orthostatic dizziness.

It is concluded that alpha-blockade is beneficial in Raynaud's syndrome and that additional beta-blockade counteracts the alpha-blocker side-effect fluid retention, reduces the heart rate and thus may prevent alpha-blocker induced tachycardia, and that it does not cause hypotension.

3.1. Introduction

In a double-blind single dose study we previously demonstrated a favorable effect of the alpha-adrenoceptor blocker phenoxybenzamine in Raynaud's syndrome [1]. This finding was consistent with earlier

21

reported uncontrolled open studies [2–6]. However, no double-blind studies on chronic alpha-blockade have been reported so far in this condition.

In our previous study [1], some of the side-effects of alpha-blockade appeared to be prevented by the addition of a beta-blocking agent. In particular this pertained to postural dizziness, exercise-induced hypotension and tachycardia. These observations are in agreement with the recent concept that characteristic side-effects of alpha-blockade are due to indirect beta-stimulation [7]. Also the effect of a combined treatment with alpha- and beta-blockade seems to have not been studied in a controlled chronic trial in Raynaud's syndrome. Therefore, we studied the effects of treatment during 8 weeks with the alpha-blocker phenoxybenzamine alone and in combination with the beta-blocker sotalol in a double-blind crossover fashion in patients with this condition.

3.2. Subjects and Methods

SUBJECTS

Of all patients eligible for the trial thirty-two gave their informed consent. Thirty-one patients completed the trial. One woman dropped out in the first week of the trial because of intolerable nausea. There were ten men and twenty-one women. The average age was 45.2 years (19–70 years). Each patient had been examined at our outpatient clinic. Diagnoses had been established by the conventional criteria [8]. Raynaud's disease had been diagnosed in twenty patients, Raynaud's syndrome with connective tissue disease in eleven: five with systemic sclerosis, three with reumatoid arthritis, two with CREST* syndrome, one with polymyositis. The duration of the syndrome at the time of entry into the study varied from 2 to 44 years (average 7.7 years). Patients stopped any drug therapy concerning Raynaud's syndrome 8 weeks before entering the study. All patients were non-smokers or had stopped smoking since at least 12 months.

---

* CREST = Calcinosis, Raynaud, Esophageal hypomotility, Scleroderma, Teleangiectasia.

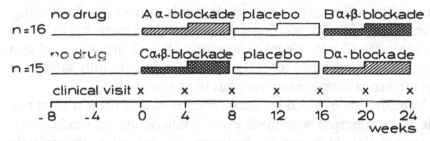

Fig. 1.   The design of the study.

DESIGN OF THE STUDY (FIGURE 1)

All patients were treated in 3 periods of 8 weeks. In the first 8 weeks period the alpha-blocker phenoxybenzamine or the combination of phenoxybenzamine plus the beta-blocker sotalol were administered in a double-blind fashion to two groups of 16 patients which were formed by block-randomization. The physician was not aware of the method of randomization. In the second 8 weeks period a placebo was administered in a single-blind way. This was considered as a wash-out period. After this wash-out a third 8 weeks period followed in which the alternate medication was given. Tablets containing one or both drugs or placebo were identical in appearance. The whole study lasted from October to April. At the start of the trial and after every 4 weeks patients were examined at our outpatient clinic. The examinations consisted of a procedure described below. Drugs were administered in oral doses, which were doubled after 4 weeks in each period: phenoxybenzamine 5 mg twice daily in the first half of the 8 weeks, and 10 mg twice daily in the second half; or the same doses of phenoxybenzamine combined with sotalol 20 mg twice daily in the first half of the 8 weeks, and 40 mg twice daily in the second half.

PROCEDURE OF EXAMINATIONS

The patient was seated quietly in a room of 24°C in order to avoid a physiological vasoconstriction [9], and a humidity of 40%. After 15 min the temperature of the volar surface of the top of the right third finger was determined by an electronic thermometer. Then, the patient's hands were placed in well-fitting plastic gloves and immersed in water of 16°C to just beyond the metacarpophalangeal joints during

5 min. The patient gently moved his hands to intensify the cooling. After taking of the gloves, finger temperature was measured as before each min for 12 min. Finger temperature after 12 min was used as a measure for temperature recovery, because in most healthy subjects at this moment a complete recovery has been reached [10].

Registrations of blood pressure (arteriosonde 1217) and heart rate (electrocardiograph) were made every 3 min during the whole period of examination. In the results, however, only the values immediately before cooling are given.

After this, a blood sample was taken for laboratory investigation including plasma creatinine, glucose, serum glutamic oxaloacetic transaminase, serum glutamic pyruvic transaminase, hemoglobin, blood morphology, C1q binding assay, complement fractions C3, C4, factor B, ANA-test. A urine analysis was performed, and body weight was recorded. The results of the C1q binding assay, the ANA-test, and the determination of C3, C4, factor B will be dealt with elsewhere. In the 8th week of the trial all patients answered without assistance of the physician a questionnaire about clinical symptoms and side-effects as compared to the before treatment situation.

ANALYSIS OF DATA

For analysis of all data obtained by objective measurements (finger temperature, body weight, blood pressure, and heart rate) the crossover design was used. To test whether this design was valid, values prior to each of the two treatments were compared with each other (Figure 1: values at A and D versus values at B and C). To trace carryover effects, values prior to any treatment were compared with the 8 weeks placebo values, separately for the patients starting on alpha-blockade and on alpha + beta-blockade (Figure 1: values at A versus B, at C versus D). To trace time-effects the same comparison was performed for the whole group (Figure 1: values at A and C versus at B and D). Other tests on carryover effects were not applied, because of the small number of patients and the small power of these kinds of tests [11, 12].

The results of 4 and 8 weeks alpha-blockade were compared with the values prior to alpha-blockade and with each other (31 patients). The same procedure was performed on alpha + beta-blockade: we analyzed effect again using the difference between posttreatment value and pretreatment value as parameter for comparison (32 patients).

TABLE I

Mean finger temperature 12 min after finger cooling prior to treatment.

1st period prior to alpha-blockade (A, $n = 16$)	$20.3 \pm 1.8°C$
3rd period prior to alpha + beta-blockade (B, $n = 16$)	$20.6 \pm 2.2°C$
1st period prior to alpha + beta-blockade (C, $n = 15$)	$20.5 \pm 1.5°C$
3rd period prior to alpha-blockade (D, $n = 15$)	$19.3 \pm 1.5°C$
1st period prior to alpha- and 3rd period prior to alpha-blockade (A + D, $n = 31$)	$19.8 \pm 1.7°C$
3rd period prior to alpha + beta-blockade and 1st period prior to alpha + beta-blockade (B + C, $n = 31$)	$20.4 \pm 1.9°C$

A, B, C, and D refer to points in Figure 1.

For analysis of clinical symptoms and side-effects a parallel group study of the first 8 weeks of the trial was performed. Decrease of complaints and appearance of side-effects after 8 weeks alpha-blockade (16 patients) were compared with the effects after 8 weeks alpha + beta-blockade (15 patients).

For statistical analysis of the crossover design Wilcoxon's test for paired data was used (two-sided, except for the results after 4 and 8 weeks treatment in comparison with the values prior to the same treatment, that were tested one-sided). For analysis of the parallel group study the Fisher's exact test for 2 × 2-table was used. We calculated 95% confidence intervals for the probabilities of decrease of complaints and appearance of side-effects. P-values of 0.05 or less were considered significant. Results are presented as mean ± standard deviation (SD).

3.3. Results

TESTS FOR THE VALIDITY OF THE CROSSOVER DESIGN (OBJECTIVE MEASUREMENT)

No significant differences were found between the values prior to each of the two treatments (Figure 1: values at A and D versus values at B and C), except for the mean finger temperature 12 min after finger cooling (Table I) that was slightly lower prior to alpha-blockade than prior to alpha + beta-blockade (19.8 ± 1.7°C versus 20.4 ± 1.9°C, $p <$ 0.05). This difference was caused by a difference between the 8 weeks placebo values (D) and the values prior to any treatment (C) in the group starting on alpha + beta-blockade (Figure 1: difference between values at D and values at C, mean decrease of -1.1 ± 2.8°C, $p < 0.01$). No other significant differences were found between 8 weeks placebo values and values prior to any treatment (Figure 1: values at A versus B, at C versus D, values at A and C versus at B and A). Despite the established slight difference in one parameter, the crossover design was considered valid, as will be discussed later. Moreover, further analysis of quantitative data have been performed using a procedure that is not influenced by differences in pretreatment values.

QUANTITATIVE EFFECTS OF ALPHA-BLOCKADE

The recovery of finger temperature 12 min after finger cooling significantly increased after 4 and after 8 weeks alpha-blockade (Table II). The 4 weeks value was significantly lower than the 8 weeks value (23.7 versus 24.5°C, $p < 0.05$). Also immediately after finger cooling (0 min) the alpha-blocker had a significant effect on finger temperature after 8 weeks treatment. This therapy did not influence blood pressure or heart rate. However, body weight significantly increased after 8 weeks treatment with a mean value of 2 kg. This was accompanied by obvious edema in 6 patients. Laboratory investigation and urine analysis did not reveal relevant differences as compared to the before-treatment situation.

QUANTITATIVE EFFECTS OF ALPHA + BETA-BLOCKADE

Also on alpha + beta-blockade there was a significant increase of finger temperature 12 min after finger cooling (Table II). Again the 4 weeks value was significantly lower than the 8 weeks value (24.1 versus 25.3°C, $p < 0.01$). This therapy did not influence blood pressure or body weight. However, heart rate significantly fell. Laboratory investigation of blood and urine did not reveal relevant differences as compared to the values before alpha + beta-blockade.

TABLE II

Influence of alpha-blockade and alpha + beta-blockade on the objectively measured variables (mean values ± S.D.).

	Alpha-Blockade		
	Before treatment $n = 31$	4 weeks treatment $n = 31$	8 weeks treatment $n = 31$
Finger temperature (°C)			
before cooling	27.2±3.6	28.1±3.0	28.6±3.2
immediately after cooling	17.9±1.0	18.5±1.2	18.8±1.1***
12 min after cooling	19.8±1.7	23.7±3.2***	24.5±3.2***
Systolic pressure (mm Hg)	127±14	128±13	125±13
Diastolic pressure (mm Hg)	85±10	85±10	83±9
Heart rate (beats/min)	75±11	77±11	77±15
Body weight (kg)	68.7±11.5	68.9±11.3	70.7±10.9*

	Alpha + Beta-Blockade		
Finger temperature (°C)			
before cooling	27.4±3.7	28.6±3.5	29.2±3.5*
immediately after cooling	'18.3±1.0	18.5±1.8	19.4±1.9**
12 min after cooling	20.4±1.9	24.1±4.8***	25.3±4.3***
Systolic pressure (mm Hg)	127±11	126±16	123±15
Diastolic pressure (mm Hg)	85±9	84±12	81±11
Heart rate (beats/min)	76±10	70±12**	70±12***
Body weight (kg)	69.0±11.7	69.5±11.5	68.5±11.0

Wilcoxon's test for paired data is used to compare 4 and 8 weeks values with the values prior to the same treatment.
* $p < 0.05$
** $p < 0.01$
*** $p < 0.001$

QUANTITATIVE EFFECTS OF ALPHA-BLOCKADE VERSUS ALPHA + BETA-BLOCKADE

Using the difference between posttreatment value and pre-treatment value as parameter for comparison between alpha-blocker and alpha + beta-blocker effects (Table III), we found that the influence of the therapies on heart rate and on body weight were significantly different:

TABLE III

Increase or decrease of objectively measured variables after alpha-blockade (posttreatment minus pretreatment values) compared with the increase or decrease after alpha + beta-blockade.

	4 Weeks Treatment		
	α-blockade $n = 31$	p	$\alpha + \beta$-blockade $n = 31$
Finger temperature (°C)			
before cooling	+0.9±2.0	NS	+1.2±3.8
immediately after cooling	+0.6±1.5	NS	+0.2±1.6
12 min after cooling	+3.9±3.0	NS	+3.7±4.5
Systolic pressure (mm Hg)	+1±10	NS	−1±17
Diastolic pressure (mm Hg)	0±7	NS	−1±11
Heart rate (beats/min)	+2±10	$p < 0.05$	−6±10
Body weight (kg)	+0.2±1.1	NS	+0.5±1.6

	8 Weeks Treatment		
	α-blockade $n = 31$	p	$\alpha + \beta$-blockade $n = 31$
Finger temperature (°C)			
before cooling	+1.4±3.5	NS	+1.8±4.5
immediately after cooling	+0.9±1.2	NS	+1.1±1.8
12 min after cooling	+4.7±3.2	NS	+4.9±4.4
Systolic pressure (mm Hg)	−2±15	NS	−4±16
Diastolic pressure (mm Hg)	−2±10	NS	+4±10
Heart rate (beats/min)	+2±10	$p < 0.05$	−6±9
Body weight (kg)	+2.0±2.0	$p < 0.05$	−0.5±2.0

on alpha + beta-blockade heart rate fell, whereas body weight did not rise. However, the influences of the therapies on finger temperature were not significantly different.

TABLE IV

Number of patients experiencing a decrease (yes) or no decrease (no) of complaints after the first 8 weeks of treatment.

Decrease of complaints	Alpha-Blocker $n = 16$			Alpha + Beta-Blocker $n = 15$		
	yes	no	95% confidence interval (%)	yes	no	95% confidence interval (%)
General	10	6	35–85	7	8	21–73
Coldness	10	6	35–85	4	11	8–55
Pain	9	7	30–80	5	10	12–62
White color	7	9	20–70	6	9	16–68
Blue color	7	9	20–70	4	11	8–55
Lesions	5	11	11–59	4	11	8–55
Duration of attacks	7	9	20–70	8	7	27–79

CLINICAL SYMPTOMS AND SIDE-EFFECTS

Table IV gives the number of patients who experienced improvement of symptoms in the first 8 weeks of the trial. The 95% confidence interval, reflecting the chance of decrease of complaints, was between 35 and 85% for the general complaints on alpha-blockade, between 21 and 73% on alpha + beta-blockade. The incidence of side effects is given in Table V, with 95% confidence intervals. The major side effects of the two medications were nasal congestion, disturbed ejaculation and potence, dry mouth, tiredness, exercise-induced and orthostatic dizziness. Other possible side-effects such as itch, loss of appetite, obstipation, diarrhea, muscle weakness, gastric pain, nausea, vomiting, blurred vision, disturbed concentration appeared to be unimportant and have, therefore, not been presented. None of the patients experienced a collapse. No significant differences between the scores for alpha-blockade and alpha + beta-blockade were found.

3.4. Discussion

The design for our study was very much determined by a number of limitations. First of all, the trial had to take place in the colder part of

TABLE V

The prevalence of side-effects after the first 8 weeks of treatment.

Side effects	Alpha-Blocker n = 16			Alpha + Beta-Blocker n = 15		
	yes	no	95% confidence interval (%)	yes	no	95% confidence interval (%)
Nasal congestion	10	6	35–85	10	5	38–88
Alcohol intolerance	2	12	2–43	2	13	4–71
Urine incontinence	5	11	11–59	5	10	12–62
Disturbed ejaculation*	4	2	22–96	2	2	7–93
Disturbed potence*	4	2	22–96	2	2	7–93
Depression	4	12	7–52	6	9	16–68
Dry mouth	8	8	25–75	11	4	45–92
Tiredness	9	7	30–80	11	4	45–92
Palpitations	5	11	11–59	2	13	2–40
Dizziness at rest	4	12	7–52	5	10	12–62
Dizziness with exercise	8	8	25–75	12	3	52–96
Orthostatic dizziness	8	8	25–75	10	5	38–88
Sleepiness	5	10	12–62	9	6	32–84

Figures relate to the number of patients showing the particular side-effects or not after 8 weeks of treatment. Some questions were not answered by all patients.
* Only for male patients.

the year, because of the seasonal character of Raynaud's syndrome and, in order to avoid bias due to the type of winter, had to be accomplished in one winter. Also, the withdrawal of previous drugs had to take place already in the colder season.

For data from objective measurements a crossover design was chosen, because of the advantage of paired comparisons between alpha-blocker and alpha + beta-blocker effects. In using a crossover design one has to deal with the potential biases of carryover effects and time effects [11]. However, adrenergic receptor blocking drugs are not curative and rather short-acting. After withdrawal of beta-blockers for 2–3 days a rebound phenomenon way even occurs [13], but then the pretreatment situation returns. Therefore, no carryover effects can be expected. Secondly, the choice of the season and the equilibration time at 24°C before each experiment should minimize any time effects.

Nevertheless, we judged it a matter of course to test for these effects and, indeed, found no difference between values prior to any treatment and 8 weeks placebo values, except for the finger temperatures 12 min after finger cooling in the patients starting on alpha + beta-blockade. However, since this difference was only small and since the values after the placebo period were even lower than those prior to any therapy, we consider the difference to have risen rather by chance than due to a carryover effect. The finding does not invalidate the over-all conclusions of this report, because effects of the two drug regimens are compared on the base of difference between posttreatment values and values prior to the same treatment and not on absolute values.

For analysis of clinical symptoms and side-effects a crossover design is very likely to be biased by psychological carryover effects [14]. Therefore, these parameters have been analyzed as a parallel group study of the first 8 weeks of the trial.

Finger skin temperature is highly related to total finger blood flow [10] and can therefore be applied to measure the disappearance of a cold-induced vasoconstriction. A standard finger cooling test serves as a model for a Raynaud's attack. We previously demonstrated that the recovery of finger temperature after a standard finger cooling test is reproducible if air temperature and smoking are controlled [9, 10] and that it is significantly lower in patients with Raynaud's syndrome than in normal subjects [1]. This was considered as evidence for the validity of this method.

The present study clearly indicates that chronic alpha-blockade improves the recovery of finger temperature after cooling. The significantly higher 12 min temperature at 8 weeks than at 4 weeks probably is more due to doubling of the dose after 4 weeks than to the longer period of treatment. The improvement of finger temperature recovery is in accordance with the decrease of complaints as registered by the questionnaire. However, with the given dose the effect was not seen in all patients. The cause for a poor response in some patients is unclear and is object of further study in our clinic.

The influence of the drug on blood pressure and heart rate in our resting, sitting, normotensive patients was negligible. However, body weight after 8 weeks of treatment increased, presumably due to fluid retention. This effect has been reported of vasodilating antihypertensive drugs. It is generally ascribed to stimulation of the renin-angiotensin-aldosterone system via arterial hypotension [15]. This mechanism seems unlikely in our patients because of absence of hypotension. However, stimulation of the above system via indirect beta-stimulation seems a more plausible explanation. In fact alpha-blocker side effects have been considered due to indirect beta-stimulation [7]. Side effects generally were mild and never, except in one case, urged patients to leave the trial. Nevertheless, some side effects were very common, e.g. nasal congestion, disturbed ejaculation and potence, dry mouth, tiredness, dizziness.

The beneficial effect of the alpha-blocker phenoxybenzamine was not reduced by the addition of the nonselective, long acting beta-blocker sotalol ($t\frac{1}{2}$ 17 hours) [16]. This is in accordance with the effects from our single dose study [1] and should encourage studies on treatment of beta-blocker induced peripheral coldness [17, 18] with alpha-blockers. Furthermore, it prevented the increase of body weight, caused by the alpha-blocker alone. This supports the above concept that the weight gain is caused by stimulation of renal beta-receptors. The beta-blocker, therefore, is of practical use in preventing fluid retention due to alpha-blockade. The addition of a beta-blocker to the alpha-blocker resulted in a lower heart rate, which supports the concept that another alpha-blocker side-effect, tachycardia, may be counteracted by beta-blockade. However, tachycardia was not observed in our trial during alpha-blockade alone. The addition of the beta-blocker to the alpha-blocker did not influence blood pressure. It is remarkable, that two potentially hypotensive drugs in these normotensive patients did not lower blood pressure.

Finally, it may be concluded that alpha-blockade is, both subjectively and objectively, effective in the majority of patients with Raynaud's syndrome. The beneficial effect improves with increase of the dose. Additional beta-blockade does not attenuate the beneficial effect. Additional beta-blockade counteracts the alpha-blocker side effect fluid retention, reduces the heart rate, and may therefore also counteract alpha-blocker induced tachycardia, and does not cause hypotension.

Acknowledgements

I am indebted to Westminster Publications INC, New York, NY, for kindly granting permission to use part of a paper previously published in ANGIOLOGY (1984; 35: 29–37).

References

1. Cleophas AJM, Fennis JFM, van 't Laar A: Alpha-and beta-blockade and beta-stimulation in Raynaud's syndrome. A double blind controlled trial. Neth J Med 25: 56 (abstract), 1982.
2. Friend DG, Edwards EA: Use of "Dibenzyline" as a vasodilator in patients with severe digital ischemia. Arch Int Med 93: 928–937, 1954.
3. Trübestein G, Sobbe A: Morbus Raynaud–Raynaud-syndrome. Med Klin 48: 1990–1995, 1974.
4. Porter JM, Snider RL, Bardana EM, Rösch J, Eidemiller LR: The diagnosis and treatment of Raynaud's phenomenon. Surgery 77: 11–23, 1975.
5. Waldo R: Prazosin relieves Raynaud's vasospasm. JAMA 241: 1037, 1979.
6. Brecht Th, Hengstmann JH: Therapeutic effects of intra-arterial phentolamine in "Raynaud's syndrome". Klin Wsch 59: 397–401, 1981.
7. Hoffman BB, Lefkowitz RJ: Alpha-adrenergic receptor subtypes. N Engl J Med 302: 1390–1396, 1980.
8. Coffman JD: Raynaud's phenomenon and disease, in Cecil Textbook of Medicine, edited by Beeson & McDermott, pp 1305–1307, 1979.
9. Cleophas AJM, Fennis JFM, van 't Laar A: Treatment of vasospastic disease with prostaglandin E₁. Br Med J 282: 1476, 1981.
10. Cleophas AJM, Fennis JFM, van 't Laar A: Finger temperature after a finger cooling test. Influence of air temperature and cigarette smoking. J Appl Physiol 52: 1167–1171, 1982.
11. Hills M, Armitage P: The two-period crossover trial. Br J Clin Pharmacol 8: 7–20, 1979.
12. Brown BW: The crossover experiment for clinical trials. Biometrics 36: 69–79, 1980.
13. Simpson FO: Hypertensive disease. In Drug Treatment, edited by Graene S. Avery, pp 655–682, 1980.
14. Barker N, Hews RJ, Huitson A, Poloniecki J: The two period crossover trial. Bias 9: 67–117, 1982.
15. Koch-Weser J: Vasodilator drugs in the treatment of hypertension. Arch Int Med 144: 1017–1027, 1974.
16. Attila M, Arstila M, Pfeffer M, Tikkanen R, Vallinkoski V, Sundquist H: Human pharmacokinetics of sotalol. Acta Pharmacol Toxicol 39: 118–128, 1976.
17. Zacharias FJ: Patient acceptibility of propranolol and the occurrence of side effects. Postgrad Med J (Suppl) 52: 87–89, 1976.
18. Marshall, AJ, Roberts CJC, Barritt DW: Raynaud's phenomenon as side effect of beta-blockers in hypertension. Br Med J 1: 1498–1499, 1976.

CHAPTER 4

A PRESSOR EFFECT OF NONSELECTIVE BETA-BLOCKERS IN DIABETICS WITH POSTURAL HYPOTENSION

Eleven patients with hyperadrenergic diabetic postural hypotension and vagal neuropathy were treated in a double-blind, placebo-controlled study with different beta-agonists and antagonists. A single dose of the $beta_2$-agonist terbutaline (5 mg) and the $beta_{1+2}$-agonist orciprenaline (10 mg) did not reduce the fall in systolic pressure on standing up, despite a significant increase in both supine and standing heart rates. The $beta_1$-antagonist with intrinsic sympathicomimetic activity (ISA) acebutolol (200 mg) and the $beta_1$-antagonist metoprolol (50 mg) did not influence the fall in systolic pressure either, despite a significant decrease in supine and standing heart rates and disappearance of increase in heart rate on standing up. Only the $beta_{1+2}$-antagonist propranolol and the $beta_{1+2}$-antagonist with ISA pindolol (5 mg) could significantly reduce or practically abolish the fall in systolic and diastolic pressure on standing up. This was accompanied by a slight decrease of heart rates and disappearance of difference between supine and standing heart rates, as seen with the other beta-antagonists. Thus, only $beta_2$-blockade reduced or abolished the fall in systolic pressure on standing up in our patients. These data were confirmed by a three-week crossover trial in 10 of these patients.

4.1. Introduction

Beta-adrenergic receptor antagonists have previously been found beneficial in subjects with postural hypotension due to sympathetic denervation. This beneficial effect may be due to intrinsic sympathicomimetic activity (ISA) on the heart [1] or to enhancement of alpha-adrenergic vasoconstriction [2] in these patients, who probably have low receptor occupancy. The present study was originally designed, not to further

34

test these hypotheses, but simply to study whether these beneficial effects would be found even when tests would be performed in a larger group of patients in a double-blind, placebo-controlled regimen. Therefore we selected patients with type I diabetes with symptoms of postural hypotension. When tested for autonomic neuropathy, however, these patients showed largely elevated levels of supine and standing plasma catecholamine concentrations. This contrasted with the low level of plasma catecholamine concentrations generally found in the previously described subjects, and therefore our patients theoretically would not benefit from beta-adrenergic receptor drugs. However, because their symptoms were the same and because we suspected that other mechanisms may play a role as well, e.g., prevention of beta-adrenergic vasodilation, we decided to perform our study. We then found out that diabetics with symptoms of postural hypotension, accompanied by vagal neuropathy and elevated levels of plasma catecholamine concentrations, can be beneficially influenced by nonselective beta-blockers.

4.2. Subjects and Methods

SUBJECTS

Twelve patients who had given their informed consent participated in the study. Each patient had been examined at our outpatient clinic. Criteria for selection were:

1. At least diabetes type I for ten years or more.
2. Symptoms of dizziness and collapses or near-collapses.
3. Preferably other symptoms of autonomic neuropathy, e.g., delayed gastric emptying, bladder atony, abnormal sweating, unawareness of hypoglycemic episodes.
4. A fall of mean arterial pressure (calculated by adding one third of the pulse pressure to the diastolic pressure) of at least 10 mm Hg [3] measured at one or more visits at the outpatient clinic.

Eleven patients completed trial 1 (7 men, 4 women), and 10 trial 2. Two patients dropped out, 1 because of reluctance, 1 because of a cold. Table I enumerates the clinical data. Four patients had proliferative, 5 had background retinopathy.

TABLE I

Clinical data and tests for vagal and sympathetic neuropathy in diabetic subjects with symptoms of postural hypotension (n = 11).

Mean age	55.1 years (28–79)
Duration of diabetes	19.6 years (10–38)
Glycosylated haemoglobin (%)	11.3 (8.1–14.2)
Retinopathy	9/10
Proteinuria	8/11
Symptomatic autonomic neuropathy	7/11
Daily insulin dose (IU)	67 (40–100)
Heart rate changes during forced breathing	
< 5 beats/min	11/11
Absence of immediate cardioacceleration on standing up	11/11
Absence of immediate cardioacceleration on handgrip	11/11
Absence of cardioacceleration in phase II and III and cardiodeceleration in phase V of the Valsalva maneuver	7/7
Absence of increase in heart rate after 1 min standing	1/11
Absence of increase in heart rate after 2 min standing	1/11

Creatinine clearance was < 100 ml/min in 5 patients. Patients were told to stop beta-blockers six weeks before entering the study. Nobody used methyldopa.

Patients were tested for autonomic neuropathy according to the methods of Wieling et al. [4], by measuring heart rate changes induced by forced breathing, standing, handgrip, and the Valsalva maneuver. Heart rate was continuously measured by an electrocardiograph at a paper speed of 50 mm/sec. Plasma catecholamine concentrations were measured by a sensitive radio-enzymatic technique [5]. Blood was drawn through an indwelling intravenous needle after thirty minutes with the patient in a supine position and after ten minutes with patient standing.

PROCEDURE OF TRIAL TESTS

We recorded supine and standing blood pressures and heart rates. Registrations of supine blood pressures and heart rates were made every minute during five minutes. Then the patients were told to stand, and blood pressure and heart rate were measured again for two minutes. In the results, however, the values immediately before standing and one minute after standing are used, according to the method of Wieling [6].

DESIGN OF TRIAL 1, A DOUBLE-BLIND, PLACEBO-CONTROLLED, SINGLE-DOSE STUDY

In 11 patients, seven tests were performed at intervals of four days. Drugs or placebo were administered orally in a single dose after an overnight fast, at 7 a.m. After ninety minutes the test started. In the meantime eating or drinking or administration of insulin was not allowed.

All patients received in random order and in a double-blind fashion the following medications: a placebo, terbutaline 5 mg, orciprenaline 10 mg, acebutolol 200 mg, metoprolol 50 mg, propranolol 40 mg, and pindolol 5 mg.

DESIGN OF TRIAL 2, A DOUBLE-BLIND, PLACEBO-CONTROLLED, CROSSOVER STUDY (THREE WEEKS)

Ten patients were treated in three periods of one week. They were divided into two groups by block randomization. During the first week period there was a single-blind placebo period (placebo tablets three times daily). Placebo tablets and pindolol tablets were similar in appearance. During the second week, one group received pindolol tablets 5 mg three times daily, the other again placebo tablets. Medications were given in a double-blind manner. Eventually there was a one-week period in which the alternate medication was given, again in a double-blind manner.

Patients were examined at the outpatient clinic every week. After the trial test as described above, patients answered a questionnaire about symptoms, and cardiac output was measured in the supine position according to the method of Teichholz [7], by use of an echocardiograph.

The crossover design was considered valid [8] because only the values of the placebos given prior to pindolol were used.

STATISTICAL ANALYSIS

For statistical analysis, Wilcoxon's test for paired or unpaired data was used, for binary data, the chi-square test.

4.3. Results

TESTS OF AUTONOMIC FUNCTION

All patients showed a heart rate change during forced breathing of < 5 beats/min and absence of immediate heart rate changes on standing up and handgrip, indicating efferent vagal dysfunction. This was confirmed by absence of immediate heart rate changes during the Valsalva maneuvers in 7 patients who could adequately perform this maneuver. In only 1 patient was a sympathetic efferent lesion found, as demonstrated by absence of increase in heart rate after one minute and after two minutes of standing. The supine and standing plasma noradrenaline levels of 2.77 and 5.24 nmol/liter, respectively, in this patient indicate that this sympathetic efferent lesion was only partial. The increase in heart rate, after one and two minutes of standing, of between 8 and 20 beats/minute in the remaining 10 patients and the largely elevated plasma catecholamine concentrations in all patients (Table II) indicate that the efferent sympathetic function generally was fairly intact. So our patients had dysfunction of vagal efferents, with fairly intact sympathetic efferents and elevated levels of plasma catecholamines.

TRIAL 1

In Figure 1, mean supine and standing blood pressures and heart rates on placebo and on medications are compared with each other. On placebo, standing caused a significant fall in systolic and diastolic pressure, and heart rate significantly increased. The $beta_2$-agonist terbutaline and the $beta_{1+2}$-agonist orciprenaline did not reduce the fall in systolic pressure on standing up, despite a significant increase in both supine and

TABLE II

Supine and standing plasma catecholamine concentrations in diabetic subjects with symptoms of postural hypotension ($n = 11$). Numbers in parentheses are the values of normal subjects ($n = 10$), (mean ± SE).

	Supine	Standing
Noradrenaline	2.7±0.6	6.3±1.2
(nmol/lite)	(1.8±0.2)	(3.3±0.3)**
Adrenaline	0.53±0.16	3.24±1.9
(nmol/liter)	(0.09±0.01)***	(0.17±0.03)(*)
Dopamine	0.55±0.18	1.05±0.30
(nmol/liter)	(0.19±0.03)*	(0.25±0.05)***

Probabilities relate to differences between patients and normal subjects.
(*) $0.05 < p < 0.1$.
* $p < 0.05$.
** $p < 0.02$.
*** $p < 0.01$.

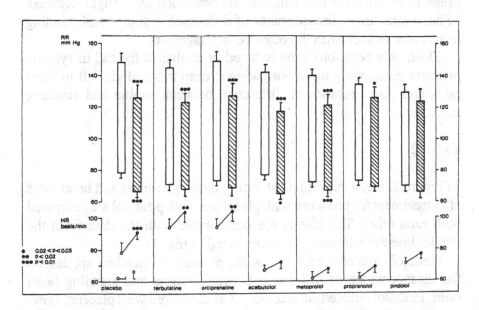

Fig. 1. Comparisons of supine and standing blood pressures and heart rates on placebo and medications (mean ± SE) in diabetics with symptoms of postural hypotension ($n = 11$). Probabilities relate to the differences between supine and standing values.

TABLE III

Effects of taking pindolol 15 mg/day for seven days on supine hemodynamic variables (mean ± SE).

	Before pindolol	p	After pindolol
Mean arterial pressure (mm Hg)	113±6	NS	108±6
Heart rate (beats/min)	84±4	NS	79±1
Cardiac output (liter/min)	5.27±0.95	NS	3.77±0.53
Stroke volume (ml)	62.7±11.5	NS	47.7±6.9

standing heart rates ($p < 0.01$). The beta$_1$-antagonist with ISA acebutolol and the beta$_1$-antagonist metoprolol did not influence the fall in systolic pressure on standing up either, despite a significant decrease in supine and standing heart rates ($p < 0.01$) and the disappearance of increase in heart rate on standing up. Only the beta$_{1+2}$-antagonist propranolol and the beta$_{1+2}$-antagonist with ISA pindolol could significantly reduce or practically abolish the fall in systolic and diastolic pressure on standing up. This was accompanied by a slight decrease of heart rates and a disappearance of difference in supine and standing heart rates, as seen with the other beta-antagonists.

Thus, only beta$_2$-blockade reduced or abolished the fall in systolic pressure on standing up in our patients, despite the slight fall in heart rates and disappearance of difference between supine and standing heart rates.

Trial 2

In Figure 2, mean supine and standing blood pressures and heart rates after treatment for one week with placebo or with pindolol are compared with each other. The effects are comparable with the data from the single-dose experiments as demonstrated in trial 1.

Pindolol reduced the fall in systolic pressure on standing up, despite the disappearance of difference between supine and standing heart rates. Pindolol reduced cardiac output as compared with placebo; however, the difference was not statistically significant (Table III). Table IV enumerates the patients who had complaints (yes or no) during placebo in the left two columns and during pindolol in the right two columns.

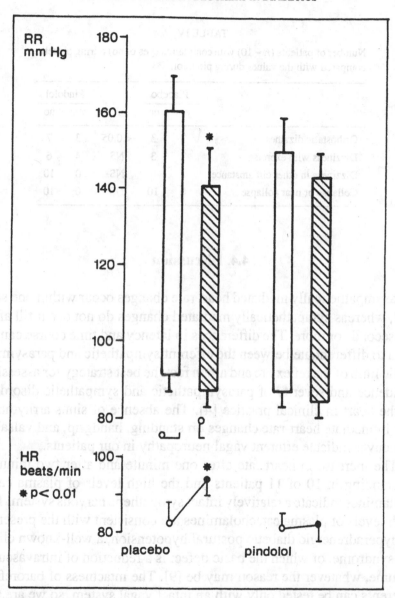

Fig. 2. Comparisons of supine and standing blood pressures and heart rates on placebo and on pindolol (mean ± SE) in diabetics with symptoms of postural hypotension ($n = 10$) in a three-week crossover trial. Probabilities relate to the differences between supine and standing values.

Seven of 10 patients experienced orthostatic dizziness during placebo. During pindolol only 3 patients were dizzy on standing. This number is significantly lower than the placebo value.

TABLE IV

Number of patients ($n = 10$) with complaints (yes or no) during placebo compared with the values during pindolol.

| | Placebo | | | Pindolol | |
	yes	no	P	yes	no
Orthostatic dizziness	7	3	< 0.05	3	7
Dizziness with exercise	7	3	NS	4	6
Dizziness in other circumstances	2	8	NS	0	10
Collapse or near collapse	0	10	NS	0	10

4.4. Discussion

Parasympathetically mediated heart rate changes occur within one second, whereas sympathetically mediated changes do not occur till after ten seconds or more. The differences in latency and time course can be used to differentiate between the efferent sympathetic and parasympathetic limb of the reflex arc and are in fact the best strategy for assessing incidence and severity of parasympathetic and sympathetic disorders of the heart in clinical practice [4]. The absence of sinus arrhythmia and immediate heart-rate changes on standing, handgrip, and valsalva maneuver indicate efferent vagal neuropathy in our patients.

The increase in heart rate after one minute and after two minutes of standing in 10 of 11 patients and the high levels of plasma catecholamines indicate a relatively intact sympathetic nervous system. The high levels of plasma catecholamines are consistent with the presence of hyperadrenergic diabetic postural hypotension, a well-known clinical syndrome, of which the basic defect is a reduction of intravascular volume, whatever the reason may be [9]. The intactness of baroreflex afferents can be tested only with an intact vagal system, so we are not informed about that. Hence, our patients suffered from vagal neuropathy and the syndrome of hyperadrenergic diabetic postural hypotension. Previously, beta-antagonists have been found beneficial in subjects with postural hypotension due to sympathetic denervation. This beneficial effect may be due to intrinsic sympathicomimetic activity on the heart, causing a supine pressure reserve high enough to prevent a large fall in blood pressure on standing up [1], or to enhancement of residual alpha vasoconstrictor activity by blocking beta-receptors for circulating catecholamines [2]. The first mechanism cannot be responsible in our patients, since ISA without beta$_2$-blockade did not cause benefit. Moreover, pindolol did not improve cardiac output, as it did in sympathetically denervated patients [1]. The second mechanism cannot be responsible in our patients either, since they had, not low, but largely elevated levels of circulating catecholamines. These elevated levels will not only stimulate alpha-receptor vasoconstriction but also beta-receptor vasodilation. A mechanism by which beta$_2$-blockers may beneficially influence postural hypotension in our patients may be prevention of beta$_2$-mediated vasodilation.

In conclusion, nonselective beta-blockade largely diminished the fall in systolic pressure on standing up in diabetics with hyperadrenergic postural hypotension and vagal neuropathy. Clinical symptoms were also alleviated by this medication. Prevention of beta$_2$-mediated vasodilation may play a role in this beneficial effect.

Acknowledgements

Measurements of plasma catecholamine concentrations were performed by Dr. J Odink, TNO-Laboratories, Zeist, The Netherlands.

I am indebted to Westminster Publications INC., New York, NY, for kindly granting permission to use part of a paper previously published in ANGIOLOGY (1986; 37: 855–862).

References

1. Man in 't Veld AJ, Schalekamp MADH: Pindolol acts as a beta-adrenoceptor agonist in orthostatic hypotension: Therapeutic implications. Br Med J 282: 929–931, 1981.
2. Chobanian AV, et al.: Use of propranolol in the treatment of idiopathic orthostatic hypotension. Trans Assoc Am Physicians 90: 324–334, 1977.
3. Plum F: Orthostatic hypotension. In: Cecil-Loeb Textbook of Medicine, ed. by Beeson PB, McDermott W., Philadelphia WB, Saunders CO, p 1928, 1979.
4. Wieling W, et al.: Assessment of methods to estimate impairment of vagal and sympathetic innervation of the heart in diabetic autonomic neuropathy. Neth J Med 28: 383–392, 1985.
5. Peuler JD, Hohnson GA: A sensitive radio-enzymatic assay for catecholamines in tissues and plasma. Life Sci 21: 625–636, 1977.
6. Wieling W, et al.: Reflex control heart rate in normal subjects in relation to age: A data base for cardiac vagal neuropathy. Diabetologia 22: 163–166, 1982.

7. Teichholz LE, et al.: Problems in echocardiographic volume determinations: Echocardiographic-angiographic correlations in the presence or absence of asynergy. Am J Cardiol 37: 7–11, 1976.
8. Cleophas TJM: Statistical concepts fundamental to investigations. N Engl J Med 313: 1026, 1985.
9. Cryer PE: Disorders of sympathetic neural function in human diabetes mellitus: Hypoadrenergic and hyperadrenergic postural hypotension. Metab Clin Exp 29: 1186–1189, 1980.

CHAPTER 5

A PRESSOR EFFECT OF NONSELECTIVE
BETA-BLOCKERS DURING ACUTE HOSPITALIZATION

Pressor effects of noncardioselective beta-blockers have been demonstrated in situations of increased sympathetic activity; however, data are limited and the clinical significance of this finding is in doubt. This chapter reports a study performed in my department to supply data about the effect of noncardioselective beta-blockers on the stress of acute hospitalization. Of 2,989 patients acutely admitted to a 50-bed unit of general internal medicine in a 647-bed teaching hospital, 234 had used beta-blockers without intrinsic sympathicomimetic activity (ISA) for at least six weeks because of mild hypertension; 199 were evaluable, 56 using nonselective, 143 using selective beta-blockers. The authors found a marked pressor effect of noncardioselective beta-blockers as compared with selective (mean arterial pressure 125 versus 102 mm Hg, $p < 0.001$). In the patients who could continue their outpatient medication this effect could be attributed to an over-all increase of total peripheral resistance and disappeared within five days of admission. In the patients admitted because of unstable angina pectoris (nonselective $n = 15$, selective $n = 48$) myocardial oxygen demand as estimated by the double-product (systolic blood pressure × heart rate) was significantly higher in the nonselective group (12,926 versus 9,581 mm Hg.beats/min, $p < 0.01$). The present study supports the need for more controlled data to determine the ultimate place of noncardioselective beta-blockers in situations of increased sympathetic activity.

5.1. Introduction

About 60% of the beta-blockers are prescribed for the treatment of hypertension. In Europe 35% of the hypertensive patients receive beta-blockers today. In the United States this number is approximately 25% [1]. Despite their popularity it is known that their hypotensive activity is sometimes small or even absent [2]. Pressor effects have

45

been described, especially with the so-called noncardioselective beta-blockers. They occur mainly in situations of increased sympathetic activity and have been ascribed to alpha-receptor-mediated vasoconstriction unopposed by beta-2-receptor-mediated vasodilation. They have been demonstrated during infusion of epinephrine and by the use of other stress models in more than fifty papers, recently reviewed by us [3]. However, data on the influence of daily life stress on this mechanism are scarce and its clinical significance is, therefore, in doubt. The implication that cardioselective beta-blockers would not be pressors, is certainly not well documented. The present study was performed to supply data about the effect of both noncardioselective and cardioselective beta-blockers on the stress of acute hospitalization. We found a marked pressor effect of noncardioselective beta-blockers as compared with selective.

5.2. Patients and Methods

We conducted a prospective study at a 50-bed unit of general internal medicine at the Department of Medicine of the Merwede Hospital, a 647-bed teaching hospital during thirty-six months between September, 1983, and September, 1986. In this period 2,989 patients were acutely admitted to this unit. We identified 234 patients with mild hypertension who had been treated at our outpatient clinic for more than four weeks with at least 80 mg propranolol daily or equipotent doses of other beta-blockers without ISA and, except for diuretics (25 mg chlorthalidone or 40 mg furosemide daily, which are standard diuretic therapies at our department) and short-acting sublingual nitrates (0.4–1.0 mg tablets of nitroglycerin), used no other hypotensive agents. Excluded from further because of hemodynamic instability were patients with acute myocardial infarction (6 patients), shock (4 patients), gastrointestinal bleeding (3 patients), and tachycardia (i.e., a heart rate > 140 beats/min, 16 patients). Excluded for the sake of symmetry (preference for cardioselective blockers) were patients with chronic obstructive pulmonary disease (COPD) (6 patients). The remaining 199 patients had been admitted because of different types of emergencies (Table I). Patients requiring nitroglycerin at the time of entry were not encountered in this study; 56 had been treated with a noncardioselective beta-blocker, 143 with a selective.

TABLE I

Patients' characteristics in the two study groups.

	Nonselective ($n = 56$)	P[@]
Male/female	21/35	NS
Mean age (range)	67.8 years (37–82)	NS
Years of hypertension (range)	11.4 years (0.4–22)	NS
Number of patients taking diuretics	15 (26%)	NS
Number of patients taking sublingual nitrates	16 (29%)	NS
Last visit to the outpatient clinic (range)	8.0 weeks (3–14)	NS
Mean daily dose of beta-blocker	propranolol 170 mg	NS[*]
(range)	(80–360) $n = 55$	
	sotalol 80 mg $n = 1$	
Type of emergency		
Unstable angina pectoris	15 (27%)	NS
Cardiac failure	9 (16%)	NS
Unstable diabetes mellitus	4 (7%)	NS
Nonsurgical abdominal symptoms	8 (14%)	NS
Peripheral vascular disease	13 (23%)	NS
Other	7 (13%)	NS
	Selective ($n = 143$)	
Male/female	64/79	
Mean age (range)	65.2 years (30–84)	
Years of hypertension (range)	14.0 years (0.6–35)	
Number of patients taking diuretics	31 (22%)	
Number of patients taking sublingual nitrates	46 (32%)	
Last visit to the outpatient clinic (range)	6.9 weeks (3–16)	
Mean daily dose of beta-blocker metoprolol	183 mg	
(range)	(100–400) $n = 94$	
	atenolol 106 mg	
	(50–200) $n = 49$	
Type of emergency		
Unstable angina pectoris	48 (34%)	
Cardiac failure	24 (17%)	
Unstable diabetes mellitus	10 (7%)	
Nonsurgical abdominal symptoms	19 (13%)	
Peripheral vascular disease	18 (13%)	
Other	24 (17%)	

[*] 80 mg propranolol was considered equipotent to 80 mg sotalol, 100 mg metoprolol, or 50 mg atenolol.
[@] nonselective versus selective beta-blockers.

As a standard procedure all patients or their relatives answered, immediately after admission to our unit, a questionnaire about their clinical symptoms and medical history, and supine blood pressure and heart rate were measured by a registered nurse. (The emergency room may expose the patients to a higher level of stress than the bed at the unit fifteen to thirty minutes later. However, after stress it may take thirty minutes or more before circulating catecholamines stop rising [4]. These data, including the blood pressures, were then checked within five to ten minutes by the attending physicians and corrected by them if not accurate (5 patients). After that the data were compared with the outpatient clinic data (hypertensive patients are always measured in the supine position at our outpatient clinic). It was decided to continue outpatient medications whenever there were no contraindications. Of the 56 patients taking noncardioselective beta-blockers, 20 could continue and did not need additional vasoactive drugs. They were enrolled in a regimen of blood pressure and heart rate measurements every one to two hours for five days and measurements of urine levels of metanephrines and of supine cardiac output by use of serial M mode echocardiograms with a 5 megahertz transducer according to Teichholz [5]. Of the 143 patients using selective blockers, 56 could continue their medication. The first 20 of them were studied similarly and served as controls for the 20 patients using noncardioselective blockers. The study was approved by our institutional ethical review committee. For statistical analysis Student's T-tests or the chi-square test were used; $P < 0.05$ was considered significant.

5.3. Results

Table I gives the patients' characteristics. No significant differences between the two study groups appeared, though the selective group was essentially larger, perhaps reflecting the house staff's customs. Table II gives the hemodynamic data of the two study groups during the last outpatient clinic visit and during the acute admission. Acute admission significantly increased systolic and diastolic blood pressure in the nonselective group but not in the selective. Comparisons between the two groups showed no differences in the outpatient clinic data. However, during acute admission systolic and diastolic blood pressure were significantly higher in the nonselective group than in the selective

TABLE II

Blood pressures and heart rates in the two study groups measured during the last visit to the outpatient clinic and during acute admission to hospital (mean ± SE).

| | Nonselective $n = 56$ | |
	Outpatient Clinic	Acute Admission
Systolic blood pressure (mm Hg)	146±3	173±4*
Mean arterial pressure (mm Hg)	104±3	125±3*
Diastolic blood pressure (mm Hg)	83±2	101±2*
Heart rate (beats/min)	67±2	73±2(*)

| | Selective $n = 143$ | |
	Outpatient Clinic	Acute Admission
Systolic blood pressure (mm Hg)	142±3	140±2
Mean arterial pressure (mm Hg)	103±2	102±2
Diastolic blood pressure (mm Hg)	82±2	84±1
Heart rate (beats/min)	70±1	71±1

(*) $0.05 < p < 0.10$, acute admission versus outpatient clinic.
* $p < 0.001$, acute admission versus outpatient clinic.

($p < 0.001$). Heart rate did not differ between the two groups, suggesting that the doses, as estimated by their chonotropic effect, were equipotent. In the patients admitted because of unstable angina pectoris, mean age and sex distribution were not significantly different between the nonselective and selective group. However, the myocardial oxygen demand as estimated by the double-product was significantly higher in the nonselective group (12,926 versus 9,581 mm Hg.beats/min, $p < 0.01$, Figure 1).

In the patients who could continue their medication and did not need additional vasoactive drugs, sex distribution and mean age were not significantly different between the nonselective patients and their selective controls. Their characteristics are shown in Table III. Only patients with noncardiac emergencies were available for this part of the study, since new vasoactive drugs were generally instituted in the remaining patients. The generally slightly elevated twenty-four hour excretions of metanephrines during the first day of admission (Table III) indicated that the acute hospitalization indeed produced a significant

TABLE III

Characteristics of the patients who could continue their outpatient medication and did not need additional vasoactive drugs.

	Nonselective (n = 20)	P@
Male/female	12/8	NS
Mean age (range)	69.9 years (37–82)	NS
Years of hypertension (range)	11.2 years (0.4–20)	NS
Mean daily dose of beta-blocker propranolol	158 mg	NS*
(range)	(80–240) n = 20	
Number of patients using diuretics	4 (20%)	NS
Number of patients using sublingual nitrates	0 (0%)	NS
Types of emergency		
Unstable diabetes mellitus	3 (15%)	NS
Nonsurgical abdominal symptoms	7 (35%)	NS
Peripheral vascular disease	3 (15%)	NS
Other	7 (35%)	NS
Mean 24-hour excretion of		
metanephrines on the first day	3.1 mmol/24 hours	NS
of admission (range)**	(1.4–6.0)	

	Selective (n = 20)
Male/female	9/11
Mean age (range)	69.5 years (54–84)
Years of hypertension (range)	12.9 years (1–28)
Mean daily dose of beta-blocker (range)	metoprolol 203 mg
	(100–300) n = 10
	atenolol 95 mg
	(50–200) n = 10
Number of patients using diuretics	5 (25%)
Number of patients using sublingual nitrates	0 (0%)
Types of emergency	
Unstable diabetes mellitus	5 (25%)
Nonsurgical abdominal symptoms	8 (40%)
Peripheral vascular disease	4 (20%)
Other	3 (15%)
Mean 24-hour excretion of	
metanephrines on the first day	3.0 mmol/24 hours
of admission (range)**	(2.0–5.1)

* 80 mg propranolol was considered equipotent to 100 mg metoprolol or 50 mg atenolol.
** Reference range 0.006–3.8 mmol/24 hours.
@ nonselective versus selective beta-blockers.

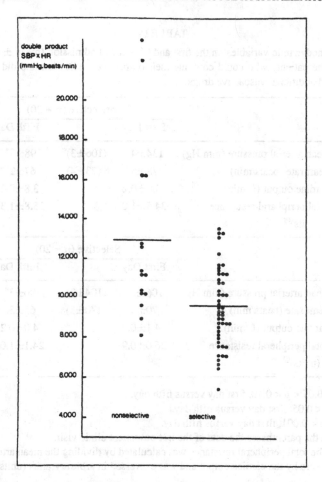

Fig. 1. Double-products of systolic blood pressure and heart rate (SBP × HR) of the patients acutely admitted because of unstable angina pectoris.

increase of neurohumoral sympathetic activity. Table IV shows the hemodynamic parameters on the first day and fifth day of admission measured during echocardiographic examination. These data reflect the data of the whole group (Table II) and show that the pressor effect is apparently due to an over-all increase of total peripheral resistance. The difference in mean arterial pressure between the nonselective and selective patients disappears within five days of admission (first day 134 versus 106 mm Hg, $p < 0.001$; fifth day 98 versus 96 mm Hg, ns; Figure 2). This effect was not accompanied by significant differences

TABLE IV

Hemodynamic variables on the first and fifth day of admission (mean ± SE) of the patients who could continue their outpatient medication and did not need additional vasoactive drugs.

	Nonselective ($n = 20$)		
	First Day		Fifth Day
Mean arterial pressure (mm Hg)	134±4	(106±3)°	98±3**
Heart rate (beats/min)	78±5	(73±4)	67±2**
Cardiac output (L/min)	3.9±0.2		3.8±0.2
Total peripheral resistance (units)@	34.5±1.0		25.8±1.3**

	Selective ($n = 20$)		
	First Day		Fifth Day
Mean arterial pressure (mm Hg)	106±3	(104±3)	96±3*
Heart rate (beats/min)	70±3	(70±3)	65±3(*)
Cardiac output (L/min)	4.1±0.2		4.0±0.2
Total peripheral resistance (units)@	26.0±0.9		24.1±1.0

(*) $0.05 < p < 0.10$, first day versus fifth day.
* $p < 0.05$, first day versus fifth day.
** $p < 0.001$, first day versus fifth day.
° In the parentheses the data of the last outpatient clinic visit.
@ The total peripheral resistance was calculated by dividing the mean arterial pressure by the cardiac output and was expressed in arbitrary units (units).

in heart rates (first day 78 versus 70 beats/min, ns; fifth day 67 versus 65 beats/min, ns; Figure 2).

Septal and posterior left ventricular wall thickness measured during echocardiography were generally not increased (data not shown), indicating that on the whole the groups did not have evidence of left ventricular hypertrophy.

5.4. Discussion

During infusion of epinephrine a pressor effect of noncardioselective, but not of cardioselective, beta-blockers can be demonstrated [6–9]. Also the pharmacologic stress of nicotine, caffeine, and insulin –

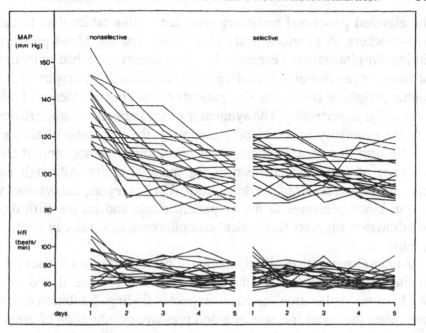

Fig. 2. Mean arterial blood pressures (MAPs) and heart rates (HRs) of the patients who could continue their outpatient medication and did not need additional vasoactive drugs.

compounds that cause a substantial rise of plasma epinephrine [10–12]' – can be used to demonstrate this pressor effect [13–28]. Finally, hypertensive crises during propranolol after withdrawal of clonidine [29–30] (alpha-2 receptor stimulation) and in untreated pheochromocytoma [31–32] have been connected with the effect. It has been ascribed to alpha-receptor-mediated vasoconstriction unopposed by beta-2-receptor-mediated vasodilation. In situations of increased sympathetic activity this mechanism may override the otherwise hypotensive properties of the nonselective blockers.

However, data on the influence of daily life stress on this mechanism are scarce. This may in part be due to the fact that stress models such as pain, loud noise, cold, etc. cause increases of catecholamines in the laboratory less than the infusion of catecholamines does [33].

This present paper demonstrates that the substantial psychological stress of acute hospitalization is accompanied by a transiently higher blood pressure and higher peripheral resistance during nonselective beta-blockade than during selective. It may be speculated that the group using nonselective blockers had more advanced hypertension and that the elevated peripheral resistance was due to this rather than to the beta-blockers. A previous study [34] found that the blood pressure during hospitalization decreased less in patients who had evidence of target organ damage, including left ventricular hypertrophy and a higher peripheral resistance. Our patients did not have evidence of left ventricular hypertrophy. The symmetry of the patients' characteristics and the symmetry of the blood pressures at the outpatient clinic and on the fifth day of admission in the two groups do not support the presence of such a mechanism in our material either. Although we have no plasma levels of the drugs studied in this report, the symmetry of the blood pressures at the outpatient clinic and on the fifth day of admission suggests that patient compliance was similar in the two groups.

Although not statistically significantly, heart rate tended to rise more in the nonselective than in the selective group (Tables II and IV). We have no explanation for this unexpected finding. Inhibition of the baroreflex due to an increase of blood pressure or inhibition of presynaptic beta-2 receptor stimulation during nonselective blockade may contribute to a decrease rather than an increase of the heart rate. A chonotropic effect of alpha-receptor stimulation seems unlikely, since the heart contains few alpha-receptors. However, because of the low level of significance the differences may have arisen by chance as well.

Our data are consistent with the Study of Drayer, who found unexpected pressor effects of propranolol in studying low renin hypertension with increased sympathetic activity [35]. Similar data were observed by Andren [36], who exposed hypertensive subjects to loud noise, a common environmental stress in industrialized countries, and found a pressor response from propranolol but not from metoprolol. Also the data of Waal-Manning [37], using mental arithmetic and handgrip as stress models; of Sangvik [38], Virtanen [39], and Nijberg [40], using handgrip; and of Atsmon [41], demonstrating a pressor effect of propranolol in psychotic patients with increased urine levels of catecholamines, are in agreement with ours. After dynamic exercise, local metabolic factors probably override the antagonistic effect on vasodilation. However, in a category with low anaerobic metabolism, namely, long-distance runners, performance was impaired with propranolol by 30% but with atenolol only by 10%. Karlson [42] attributed this effect to prevention of beta-2-receptor-mediated vasodilation. The anaerobic vasodilation may explain why the studies that use dynamic exercise as the stress model, e.g., angina pectoris studies, generally do not find differences between nonselective and selective blockers [43, 44].

Should we, because of the available data, prefer a selective to a nonselective beta-blocker to treat our patients with hypertension and angina pectoris? It should be noted that the pressor effects are usually mild. In our study mean arterial pressure was approximately 25 mm Hg higher during nonselective than during selective blockade. In the other controlled studies published till now the effect was frequently ± 10 mm Hg and has never been more than 30 mm Hg. Moreover, if we discontinue the nonselective blockers, then we discontinue the theoretical advantage of presynaptic beta-2 blockade, which has been considered one of the hypotensive mechanisms of nonselective blockers [45].

We conclude that the stress of acute hospitalization causes, in mildly hypertensive patients, a pressor effect of noncardioselective, but not of selective, beta-blockers. The current study provides data to add further support to the concept that noncardioselective beta-blockers may cause an apparent paradoxical increase in blood pressure under stressful conditions, presumably by blocking beta-2-receptor-mediated vasodilation and leaving alpha-receptor-mediated vasoconstriction intact. The clinical importance of the observations cannot be determined from the current study, although a comparative study involving patients with angina pectoris treated with a selective or nonselective beta-blocker would obviously be of interest.

Acknowledgment

We are indebted to Dr. F.H.W. Kauw, Dr. J. Meijers, and Dr. P. Tavenier for helpful discussions and to Mrs Gre Hofman and Mrs Agaath Weggers (nurses), who assisted in the study.

I am indebted to Westminster Publications INC, New York, NY, for kindly granting permission to use part of a paper previously published in ANGIOLOGY (1990; 41: 125–132).

References

1. Hefland WH: A market analyst's perspective on hypertension and its treatment. In: Hypertension and the Angiotension System: Therapeutic Approaches, ed. by Doyle AE, Bearn AG. New York: Raven Press, pp 20–24, 1984.

2. Laragh JH: Conceptual diagnostic and therapeutic dimensions of the renin system. In: Hypertension and the Angiotensin System: Therapeutic Approaches, ed. by Doyle AE, Bearn AG. New York: Raven press, p 67, 1984.

3. Cleophas TJ, Kauw FHW: Pressor responses from noncardio-selective beta-blockers. Angiology 39: 587–596, 1988.

4. Kjeldsen SE, Westheim A, Aakenson J, et al.: Plasma adrenaline and noradrenaline during orthostasis in man: The importance of arterial sampling. Scand J Clin Invest 46: 397–401, 1986.

5. Teichholz LE: Problems in echocardiographic volume determinations: Echocardiographic-angiographic correlations in the presence or absence of asynergy. Am J Cardiol 37: 7–11, 1976.

6. van Herwaarden CLA: Selective and nonselective beta-blockade in hypertension. Thesis, Nijmegen, The Netherlands, 1978.

7. Johnson G: Influence of metoprolol and propranolol on haemo-dynamic effects induced by adrenaline and physical work. Acta Pharmacol Toxicol 36 (suppl): 59–68, 1975.

8. Houben H, Thien T, de Boo T, et al.: Influence of selective and nonselective beta-adrenoceptor blockade on the haemodynamic effect of adrenaline during combined anti-hypertensive drug therapy. Clin Sci 57 (suppl): 387–389, 1979.

9. Houben H, Thien T, van 't Laar A: Effect of low-dose epinephrine infusion on haemodynamics after selective and nonselective beta-blockade in hypertension. Clin Pharmacol Ther 31: 685–690, 1982.

10. Robertson RP, Porte D: Adrenergic modulation of basal insulin secretion in man. Diabetes 22: 1–8, 1973.

11. Cryer PLE, Haymond MW, Santiago JV, et al.: Norepinephrine and epinephrine release and adrenergic mediation of smoking-associated hemodynamic and metabolic events. N Engl J Med 295: 573–577, 1976.

12. Houben H: Haemodynamic effects of stress during selective and nonselective beta-blockade. Thesis, Nijmegen, The Netherlands, 1982.

13. Trap-Jensen J, Carlsen JE, Svendsen TJL, et al.: Cardiovascular and adrenergic effects of cigarette smoking during immediate nonselective and selective beta-adrenergic blockade in humans. Eur J Clin Invest 9: 181–183, 1979.

14. Ramsay LE, Freestone S: Effects of chronic beta-blockade on the pressor response to cigarette smoking. Br J Clin Pharmacol 15: 596–597, 1983.

15. Cuspidi S, Aliprandi PL, Cavalline F: Effects of short- and long-term beta-blockade on changes in blood pressure caused by cigarette smoking in normotensive and hypertensive subjects. Drugs 25 (suppl 2): 148–149, 1983.

16. Fogari J, Parini A, Finardi G: Cardiovascular response to cigarette smoking during adrenergic block in essential hypertension. Drugs 25 (suppl 2): 149–150, 1983.

17. Brandsborg O, Christensen NJ, Galbo H, et al.: The effect of exercise, smoking and propranolol on serum gastrin in patients with duodenal ulcer and in vagotomized subjects. Scan J Clin Lab Invest 38: 441–446, 1978.

18. Westfall TC, Cipolloni PB, Edmundowics AC: Influence of propranolol on hemodynamic changes and plasma catecholamine levels following cigarette smoking and nicotine. Proc Soc Exp Biol Med 123: 174–179, 1966.

19. Freestone S, Ramsay LE: Effect of beta-blockade on the pressor response to coffee plus smoking in patients with mild hypertension. Drugs 25 (suppl): 141–145, 1983.

20. Lloyd-Mostyn RH, Oram S: Modification by propranolol of cardiovascular effects on induced hypoglycemia. Lancet 1: 1312–1315, 1979.

21. Davidson N, Corrall RJ, Shaw TR, et al.: Observations in man of hypoglycemia during selective and nonselective beta-blockade. Scott Med J 22: 69–72, 1976.

22. Sonksen PH, Brown PM, Saunders J: Metabolic effects of betaxolol during hypoglycemia and exercise in normal volunteers. In: L.E.R.S., Vol 1, ed. by Morselli PL, et al. New York: Raven Press, pp 143–155, 1983.

23. Ostman J, Aner J, Haglund K, et al.: Effect of metoprolol and alprenolol on the metabolic, hormonal, and haemodynamic responses to insulin-induced hypoglycemia in hypertensive insulin-dependent diabetics. Acta Med Scand 211: 381–385, 1982.

24. Lauridsen UB, Christensen MJ, Lyngsoe J: Effects of non-selective and beta-1 selective blockade on glucose metabolism and hormonal response during insulin-induced hypoglycemia in normal man. J Clin Endocrinol Metab 56: 876–882, 1983.

25. Kolendorf J, Aerenlund Jensen H, Holst JJ, et al.: Effects of acute selective beta-adrenergic blockade on hormonal and cardiovascular response to insulin-induced hypoglycemia in insulin-dependent diabetic patients. Scand J Clin Lab Invest 42: 69–74, 1982.

26. Pape J: Blood pressure and pulse response to insulin during nonselective and selective beta-blockade. Acta Med Scand 210 (suppl 1): 105–108, 1981.

27. Nillson OR, Karlberg BE, Soderberg A: Plasma catecholamines and cardiovascular responses to hypoglycemia in hyperthyroidism before and during treatment with metoprolol and propranolol. J Clin Endocrinol Metab 50: 906–911, 1980.

28. Ryan JR, Lacorte W, Jain A, et al.: Response of diabetics treated with atenolol or propranolol to insulin-induced hypoglycemia. Drugs 25 (suppl 2): 256–257, 1983.

29. Bailey R, Neale TJ: Rapid clonidine withdrawal with blood pressure overshoot exaggerated by beta-blockade. Br Med J 1: 1942–1943, 1976.

30. Warren SE, Ebert E, Swerdlin AH, et al.: Clonidine and propranolol paradoxical hypertension. Arch Intern Med 139: 253–257, 1979.

31. Nickerson M, Collier B: Beta-adrenergic blocking agents. In: The Pharmacological Basis of Therapeutics, ed. by Goodman LS, Gilman A. New York: MacMillan Publishing Co, pp 547–552, 1975.

32. Bravo EL, Gifford RW: Pheochromocytoma: Diagnosis, localization and management. N Engl J Med 311: 1298–1303, 1987.

33. Robertson D, Jonson GA, Robertson RM, et al.: Comperative assessment of stimuli that release neuronal and adrenomedullary catecholamines in man. Circulation 59: 637–643, 1979.

34. Nishimura H, Nishioka A, Kubo S, et al.: Multifactorial evaluation of blood pressure fall upon hospitalization in essential hypertensive patients. Clin Sci 73: 135–141, 1987.

35. Drayer JL, Keim HJ, Weber MA, et al.: Unexpected pressor response to propranolol in essential hypertension on interaction between renin, aldosterone, and sympathetic activity. Am J Med 60: 897–903, 1976.

36. Andren L, Hanssen L, Bjorkman M: Haemodynamic effects of noise exposure before and after beta-1 selective and non-selective beta-adrenoceptor blockade in patients with essential hypertension. Clin Sci 61: 89–91, 1981.

37. Waal-Manning HJ: Atenolol and three nonselective beta-blockers in hypertension. Clin Pharmacol Ther 25: 8–18, 1979.

38. Sangvik K, Stokkeland M, Lindseth EM, et al.: Circulation reaction at rest and during isometric exercise in hypertensive patients: Influence of different adrenergic beta-adrenoceptor antagonists. Pharmatherapeutica 1: 71–83, 1976.
39. Virtanen K, Janne J, Frick MH: Response of blood pressure and plasma norepinephrine to propranolol, metoprolol and clonidine during isometric exercise and dynamic exercise in hypertensive patients. Eur J Clin Pharmacol 21: 275–279, 1982.
40. Nijberg G: Blood pressure and heart rate during sustained handgrip in hypertensive patients taking placebo, a non-selective beta-blocker and a selective beta-blocker. Curr Ther Res 22: 828–838, 1977.
41. Atsmon A, Blom I, Steiner M, et al.: Further studies with propranolol in psychotic patients: Relation to initial psychiatric state, urinary catecholamines, and 3-methoxy-4-hydroglycol excretion. Psychopharmacologica 27: 249–254, 1972.
42. Karlson J: Muscle fiber composition, short-term beta-1 and beta-2 blockade and endurance exercise performance in healthy young men. Drugs 25 (suppl): 241–246, 1983.
43. Taylor SH, Silke B, Lee PS: Intravenous beta-blockade in coronary heart disease. Is cardioselectivity of intrinsic sympathicomimetic activity hemodynamically useful? N Engl J Med 306: 631–635, 1982.
44. Prida XE, Feldman RL, Hill JA, et al.: Comparison of selective and nonselective beta-adrenergic blockade on systemic and coronary hemodynamic findings in angina pectoris. Am J Cardiol 60: 244–248, 1987.
45. Langer SZ: Presynaptic receptors and their role in the regulation of transmitter release. Br J Pharmacol 60: 481–497, 1977.

CHAPTER 6

A PRESSOR EFFECT OF NONSELECTIVE
BETA-BLOCKERS DURING SURGERY UNDER
ANESTHESIA

Sixty-two patients with mild hypertension were randomly assigned to receive either no treatment, or 160 mg propranolol, or 200 mg metoprolol daily starting 1 week before elective surgery under anesthesia. The last dose was given 2 hours before anesthesia. Anesthesia consisted of induction with midazolam 2.5–5 mg followed by thiopental 250–500 mg and was maintained with 60% inspired N_2O in oxygen and 0.4% enflurane inspired. Airway carbon dioxide was monitored continuously by a CO_2 analyzer. Preoperative blood pressures were equally reduced by the two beta-blockers. During anesthesia however blood pressure further decreased in the metoprolol group but not in the propranolol group. We conclude that propranolol is less effective than metoprolol in mildly hypertensive patients during surgery under anesthesia, probably due to a pressor response from propranolol during the stress of surgery. Also, however, that the quantity of blood pressure reduction by selective beta-blockade (metoprolol) may not be needed. And that anesthesia itself is an effective means of reducing the blood pressure.

6.1. Introduction

During infusion of epinephrine a pressor effect of noncardioselective but not of cardioselective beta-blockers can be demonstrated [1, 2]. This finding supports the hypothesis that nonselective beta-blockers can cause pressor responses in situations of increased sympathetic activity due to alpha-receptor-mediated vasoconstriction unopposed by beta-2-receptor-mediated vasodilation. In situations of increased sympathetic activity this mechanism may override the otherwise hypotensive properties of nonselective beta-blockers. This hypothesis was first raised some 10 years ago and has been pursued since then by many investigators. By now 50 reports have been published. We reviewed them in an Angiology article in 1988 [3]. Many stress models have been used for example pharmacologic stress (nicotine, caffeine, insulin increase plasma epinephrine), environmental stress (loud noise), mental stress (arithmetic), physical stress (handgrip). Most of the studies did demonstrate pressor effects, but were without exception performed in laboratory settings. What about the influence of daily life stress on this pressor mechanism? In order to answer this question we recently performed two studies. The first one is entitled "A pressor effect of nonselective beta-blockers during acute hospitalization" and was published in the February issue of Angiology [4]. The present paper reports our second effort to demonstrate this pressor mechanism in daily life stress. It focuses on the stress of surgery under anesthesia. It is concluded that nonselective beta-blockade is less effective than selective in mildly hypertensive patients during surgery under anesthesia.

6.2. Patients and Methods

Seventy-five patients with mild hypertension, according to the Joint National Committee's criterion [5] (diastolic blood pressure 90–105 mm Hg, previously untreated) were randomly assigned to receive either no treatment, or 160 mg propranolol, or 200 mg metoprolol daily starting 1 week before elective surgery under anesthesia. The last dose was given 2 hours before anesthesia. 13 patients dropped out, 8 because they were not compliant with their treatment regimens, 5 because their physicians (i.e., anesthesiologists) were not. Data of the remaining 62 patients are fairly symmetric (Table I). No patient had left ventricular hypertrophy on x-ray or electrocardiogram. Anesthesia was performed by three of the authors under a strict regimen. It consisted of induction with midazolam (2.5–5 mg) followed by thiopental (250–500 mg) and was maintained with 60% inspired N_2O (nitrogene oxide) in oxygen and 0.4% enflurane inspired. Airway carbon dioxide was monitored continuously by a CO_2 analyzer, as was central venous pressure. A fall of venous pressure was corrected by increased administration of fluid. With increments of venous pressure of more than 12 cm H_2O 40 mg of furosemide was administered. Blood loss was corrected for by weighing swabs and measuring the suction bucket.

TABLE I

Patients' characteristics in the three study groups.

	Characteristics		
	No Treatment ($n = 24$)	Metoprolol ($n = 17$)	Propranolol ($n = 21$)
Male/Female	8/16	5/12	6/15
Mean age (range)	61.7 (32–75)	65.0 (36–76)	65.5 (38–80)
Signs of Left Ventricular Hypertrophy	0	0	0
Type of Surgery			
Meniscectomy	1	1	–
Anterior resection	1	–	2
Cholecystectomy	3	–	2
Osteosynthesis femur	2	–	–
Subtotal gastrectomy	2	1	–
Total hip	5	4	4
Implantation of stapes	–	–	1
Mastectomy	1	2	1
Descencus uteri	2	2	2
Excision of varicose veins	1	–	1
Hernia femoralis	–	1	1
Hysterectomy	3	1	2
TUR bladder	–	3	1
Femoro-poplit bypass	1	1	4
Strumectomy	2	1	–

All blood pressures, heart rates, and forearm blood flows, recorded by an iridium strain gauge venous occlusion plethysmograph, were measured with the patients in the supine position. Vascular resistance was calculated by dividing mean arterial pressure (diastolic blood pressure + 1/3 pulse pressure) by the forearm blood flow and was expressed in arbitrary units (units). Urine levels of metanephrines were measured on the day of surgery and the next day.

The study was approved by our institutional ethical review committee. For statistical analyses Student's T-tests or chi-square tests were

TABLE II

24-hours excretion of metanephrines (mmol/24 hours) on the day of surgery and the next day (range).

	No Treatment	Metoprolol	Propranolol
Day of Surgery	3.8 (1.3–6.1)	3.0 (1.6–5.1)	2.9 (0.8–6.7)
Next Day	0.5 (0.1–3.5)	1.2 (0.09–3.2)	0.7 (0.01–3.2)
Reference Range	0.006–3.8 mmol/24 hours		

TABLE III

Systolic blood pressures before and during surgery under anesthesia (mm Hg).

Outpatient Clinic	Pre-operative	After Intubation	10 min Anesthesia	30 min	60 min
No Treatment					
167±6(*)	161±5	167±6(*)	143±7***	153±6(*)	151±7*
Metoprolol					
165±6***	130±5	135±5	118±6**	119±6*	116±6***
Propranolol					
163±5***	129±4	139±5*	124±5	134±5	137±7(*)

(*) $0.05 < P < 0.1$ versus preoperative.
* $P < 0.05$.
** $P < 0.01$.
*** $P < 0.001$.

used; $P < 0.05$ was considered significant. Data are presented as means ± SE.

6.3. Results

Table II shows the excretions of metanephrines, which can be used as a level of sympathetic activity [4]. On the day of surgery, the range was about 1–6 mmol/24 hours which is 2–3 times higher than the reference range in all 3 groups. Next day the excretions had returned to normal levels. This indicates that surgery under anesthesia indeed can be used as a stress model. Tables III through VII show the results of the hemo-

TABLE IV

Diastolic blood pressures before and during surgery under anesthesia (mm Hg).

Outpatient Clinic	Pre-operative	After Intubation	10 min Anesthesia	30 min	60 min
No Treatment					
101±5*	91±5	89±3	84±5(*)	82±5*	86±3
Metoprolol					
97±4***	78±3	81±3	71±4(*)	72±4(*)	71±3*
Propranolol					
98±4**	82±4	83±3	74±3(*)	82±3	83±3

(*) $0.05 < P < 0.1$ versus preoperative.
* $P < 0.05$.
** $P < 0.01$.
*** $P < 0.001$.

dynamic variables in the 3 groups before and during anesthesia. Preoperative systolic blood pressures were equally reduced by the two beta-blockers (Table III). During anesthesia systolic blood pressure initially increased somewhat due to the intubation. Then it further decreased in the metoprolol group but not in the propranolol group. Anesthesia itself reduced the systolic blood pressure in the no treatment group as well by 10–15 mm Hg. A similar course was observed for the diastolic blood pressures (Table IV). Preoperative blood pressures were equally reduced by the two beta-blockers. During anesthesia a further decrease in the selective but not in the nonselective group was noted. Heart rates (Table V) were similarly reduced by the two beta-blockers although the propranolol data were consistently somewhat higher than the metoprolol; anesthesia did not markedly influence them, in either of the two groups. Forearm blood flows in the metoprolol group remained largely unchanged (Table VI). In the propranolol group, however, they tended to fall probably due to alpha-receptor-mediated vasoconstriction unopposed by beta-2-receptor-mediated vasodilation. In the no treatment group they tended to rise probably connected with beta-2-receptor-mediated vasodilation. Forearm vascular resistance (Table VII) significantly increased in the propranolol group, supporting the idea that peripheral vasoconstriction is responsible for the pressor mechanism of the nonselective beta-blockers.

TABLE V

Heart rates before and during surgery under anesthesia (beats/min).

Outpatient Clinic	Pre-operative	After Intubation	10 min Anesthesia	30 min	60 min
No Treatment					
82±4	79±3	91±4***	92±5***	87±6**	85±4*
Metoprolol					
80±3**	69±2	72±2	71±3	68±3	67±3
Propranolol					
81±3**	71±3	71±3	75±4	70±2	71±4

(*) 0.05 < P < 0.1 versus preoperative.
*   P < 0.05.
**   P < 0.01.
*** P < 0.001.

TABLE VI

Forearm blood flows before and during surgery under anesthesia (ml/100 ml tissue. min).

Outpatient Clinic	Pre-operative	10 min Anesthesia	60 min Anesthesia
No Treatment			
3.7±0.3	3.9±0.4	5.2±0.6(*)	5.3±0.5(*)
Metoprolol			
3.9±0.3	4.0±0.5	4.2±0.4	4.1±0.4
Propranolol			
4.1±0.4	3.7±0.4	3.0±0.3(*)	2.9±0.3(*)

(*) 0.05 < P < 0.1 versus preoperative.

Figure 1 gives a plot of the mean arterial pressures and heart rates in the 3 groups. The curves start immediately after intubation. Heart rates were equally reduced by the two beta-blockers. Blood pressures during metoprolol were significantly lower than during propranolol. They sometimes even went so extremely low that the anesthesiologists had to be disciplined not to interfere. Moreover, the metoprolol blood pressures were less stable and showed frequent fluctuations, probably connected in some way with the extremely low blood pressures.

TABLE VII

Forearm vascular resistances before and during surgery under anesthesia (units).

Outpatient Clinic	Pre-operative	10 min Anesthesia	60 min Anesthesia
No Treatment			
	33±4	29±3	20±4(*)	20±3(*)
Metoprolol			
	31±4	24±3	21±3	21±3
Propranolol			
	29±4	25±4	30±4	35±4*

(*) 0.05 < P < 0.1 versus preoperative.
* P < 0.05.

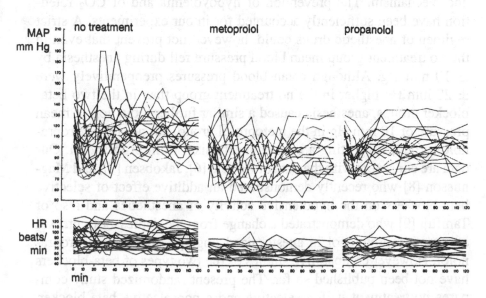

Fig. 1. Mean blood pressures and heart rates of mildly hypertensive patients during surgery under anesthesia with or without pretreatment with beta-blockers.

6.4. Discussion

A pressor response from noncardioselective beta-blockers but not from cardioselective has been demonstrated in situations of increased sympathetic activity [1–3]. This mechanism is generally ascribed to alpha-receptor-mediated vasoconstriction unopposed by beta-2-receptor-mediated vasodilation during increased sympathetic activity. Many reports did demonstrate pressor effects but were without exception performed in laboratory settings [3]. What about the influence of daily stress on this mechanism? In order to answer this question we recently performed two studies in our department. The first one is entitled "A pressor effect of nonselective beta-blockers during acute hospitalization"[4]. Of 199 hypertensive patients acutely admitted to hospital while on beta-blockers admission blood pressure was 23 mm Hg higher in the nonselective than in the selective group. The present paper reports our second effort to demonstrate this pressor mechanism in daily stress situations. It focuses on the stress of surgery under anesthesia. The increased levels of metanephrines suggest that surgery under anesthesia can indeed be used as a stress model. It is, however, a complexe situation wherein hypotension may occur from more than one mechanism. The prevention of hypovolemia and of CO_2 retention have been sufficiently accounted for in our experiments. A strict regimen of anesthetic drugs could, however, not prevent that even in the no treatment group mean blood pressure fell during anesthesia by ± 10 mm Hg. Although mean blood pressures preoperatively were ± 20 mm Hg higher in the no treatment group than in the two beta-blocker groups, anesthesia caused a similar further reduction of mean pressure of 10 mm Hg in the metoprolol group, but not in the propranolol group, suggesting a pressor mechanism from propranolol. Our data are consistent with the data of Achola [6], Jakobsen [7], and Magnusson [8] who recently demonstrated an additive effect of selective beta-blockers on the hypotensive activity of anesthetics and also of Tanifuji [9] who demonstrated a change from the depressor to pressor effect of isoproterenol in anesthesized dogs pretreated with propranolol. However comparative studies of the two types of beta-blockers have not been published so far. The present randomized study compares no treatment with a selective and a nonselective beta-blocker. We demonstrate that in spite of equipotent doses metoprolol causes a larger reduction of blood pressure during surgery under anesthesia than propranolol does. We also demonstrate, however, that the large amount of blood pressure reduction by metoprolol may not be needed and that anesthesia itself is an effective means of reducing the blood pressure. Two schools of thought exist about whether or not elective surgery in hypertensive patients should be postponed until normal blood pressure is established [10]. The current study cannot give a definitive answer to this dilemma, but the extremely low blood pressures from use of metoprolol and, in addition, the reduction of mean blood pressure in the no treatment group by 10 mm Hg support the view that there is, indeed, no need for preoperative treatment of blood pressure in this category of hypertensive patients. Although not statistically significantly, heart rate was consistently somewhat higher in the nonselective than in the selective group. We have no explanation for this puzzling finding, that was established in our previous study as well [4]. Inhibition of the baroreflex due to increase of blood pressure, or inhibition of presynaptic beta-2 receptors, or a shift from cardiac beta-1- to beta-2-receptor activity in the heart in situations of increased sympathetic activity [11] are all possibilities that should reduce the heart rate to a larger extent during propranolol than during metoprolol administration. One may speculate that propranolol prevents epinephrine from occupying vascular beta-2-receptors. More circulating epinephrine may subsequently be left to stimulate chonotropic cardiac beta-receptors. However this hypothesis is not supported by the equal levels of metanephrines in the metoprolol and propranolol group in this paper. Differences may, of course, because of their small sizes, have risen by chance.

In conclusion, the present randomized study compares no treatment with a selective and a nonselective beta-blocker in mildly hypertensive patients during surgery under anesthesia. We demonstrate that in spite of equipotent doses metoprolol causes a larger reduction of blood pressure than propranolol does. We also demonstrate, however, that the large amount of blood pressure reduction by metoprolol may not be needed, and that anesthesia itself is an effective means of reducing the blood pressure.

Acknowledgement

We are indebted to Dr. F.H. Kauw and Dr. J. Meijers for helpful suggestions and to Miss Babette Gladpootjes for expert secretarial assistance.

I am indebted to Westminster Publications INC., New York, NY, for kindly granting permission to use part of a paper previously published in ANGIOLOGY (1991; 42: 805–811).

References

1. van Herwaarden CLA: Selective and nonselective beta-blockade in hypertension. Thesis, Nijmegen, The Netherlands, 1978.
2. Johnson G: Influence of metoprolol and propranolol on haemodynamic effects induced by adrenaline and physical work. Acta Pharmacol Toxicol 36 (suppl): 59–68, 1975.
3. Cleophas TJ, Kauw FHW: Pressor responses from noncardioselective beta-blockers. Angiology 39:587–596, 1988.
4. Cleophas TJ, Stapper GJ: A pressor effect of noncardioselective beta-blockers in mildly hypertensive patients during acute hospitalization. Angiology 41: 124–132, 1990.
5. Chobanian AV: The 1988 report of the Joint National Committee on detection, evaluation, and treatment of high blood pressure. Arch Intern Med 148: 1023–1033, 1988.
6. Achola KJ, Jones MJ, Mitchell RW, et al.: Effects of beta-adrenoceptor antagonism on the cardiovascular and catecholamine responses to tracheal intubation. Anaesthesia 43: 433–436, 1988.
7. Jakobsen CJ, Grabe N, Christensen B: Metoprolol decreases the amount of halothane required to general anaesthesia. Brit J Anaesth 58: 261–266, 1986.
8. Magnusson J, Thulin T, Werner O, et al.: Haemodynamic effects of pretreatment with metoprolol in hypertensive patients undergoing surgery. Brit J Anaesth 58: 251–260, 1986.
9. Tanifuji Y, Eger EJ: Effect of isoproterenol and propranolol on halothane MAC in dogs. Anaesthesia and Analgesia 55: 383–387, 1976.
10. Merin RG. Anaesthetic implications of concurrent diseases. In: Anaesthesia, ed. by Miller RD, New York: Churchill Livingstone, p 270, 1986.
11. Moromura S: On the physiologic role of beta-2-adrenoceptors in the human heart: in vitro and in vivo studies. Am Heart J 119: 608–610, 1990.

CHAPTER 7

A PRESSOR EFFECT OF NONSELECTIVE
BETA-BLOCKERS IN UNSTABLE ANGINA PECTORIS

Background – Celiprolol, a novel beta-blocker, may be more effective than propranolol in unstable angina pectoris because of both its beta-1-receptor selectivity and its vasodilatory property.

Methods – 53 Patients with angiographic coronary artery disease but uncompromised left ventricular function and with electrocardiographically documented recurrent angina pectoris in spite of bed rest, aspirin, and repeated sublingual administration of nitroglycerin (NTG) were randomized for 1 week of treatment with equipotent doses of either the non-selective beta-blocker propranolol (80 mg dd) or the selective beta-blocker with beta-2-agonistic property celiprolol (200 mg dd).

Results – Angina frequency was higher in the propranolol group ($P < 0.01$), whereas myocardial oxygen demand as estimated by the double-product (double-product = SBP × HR, systolic blood pressure x heart rate) was equally reduced by the two beta-blockers. Forearm blood flow was essentially higher in the celiprolol group ($p < 0.001$). A stepwise logistic regression analysis showed that the beneficial effects of the beta-blockers were largely dependent on their effect on peripheral flow, in addition to reduction of the double-product.

Conclusions – 1. Both celiprolol and propranolol largely reduce angina pectoris frequency in unstable angina pectoris. 2. Celiprolol contributes to nearly complete relief in three times as many patients as propranolol; after adjustment for double-product or for systolic blood pressure plus heart rate it did so in even 8 times as many patients. 3. The similar effects of the two compounds on the double-product, and the essentially different effects on peripheral flow support the theory that celiprolol exerts its beneficial effect to a large extent through its vasodilatory property.

69

7.1. Introduction

A large body of evidence has shown that patients with unstable angina pectoris can be stabilized with beta-blockers in addition to bedrest and nitrates. After the large randomized trials of the mid 80's [1–3] involving many thousands of patients, beta-blockers have been routinely used for the treatment of unstable angina and impending infarction and even for the prevention of recurrence afterwards. The beneficial effect is probably mainly due to decrease of systolic blood pressure and heart rate. The double product, which is the product of systolic blood pressure and heart rate is a direct estimate of myocardial oxygen demand. It is largely reduced by beta-blockers. The present paper tries to test two hypotheses. First, we hypothesized that a beta-1-selective blocker would be more effective in controlling unstable angina than a nonselective blocker because unstable angina and infarction are stressful situations and nonselective blockers can cause paradoxical pressor effects during stress [4–7]. This would be disadvantageous with respect to the double-product. Secondly, we hypothesized that a beta-blocker with a vasodilatory property would be more effective than a beta-blocker without such property, because vasodilation causes preload and afterload reduction (reduced ventricular filling pressure and reduced peripheral resistance). For that reason vasodilators are currently increasingly being used in unstable angina and impending infarction with or without cardiac failure [8].

Celiprolol is a novel beta-1 selective beta-blocker with additional vasodilator properties. Propranolol is a standard nonselective beta-blocker. The first objective of this study was to determine whether celiprolol would be more effective than propranolol in controlling unstable angina pectoris. Secondly, we assessed what would be the dependent and independent variables of persistent angina pectoris in spite of the treatments given. For that purpose a multivariate analysis was applied.

7.2. Patients and Methods

Patients were recruited from the admissions to our institution because of crescendo angina pectoris between April 1992 and July 1993. Patients with ST-segment depression of more than 1 mm during pain were initially treated with bedrest, iv NTG, and aspirin 300 mg daily. Once the pain was controlled and myocardial infarction was excluded intravenous NTG was replaced by short acting sublingual nitrates ad libitum and patients were reactivated. In the patients with recurrent angina pectoris during reactivation coronary angiography was performed. 68 patients with one or more stenoses of more than 50% were considered for further study. All were in sinus rhythm and without clinical or radiographic signs of left ventricular failure. None had a history of chronic obstructive pulmonary disease or myocardial infarction. Informed consent was given by all patients, and the investigation was approved by the hospital ethics committee. They were randomized by block randomization in a double blind fashion for treatment with equipotent oral doses of celiprolol (200 mg once daily) or propranolol (80 mg once daily). According to others [9–11], we considered these doses equipotent because of their abilities to inhibit the beta-agonistic effects of isoproterenol equally. Because this was a clinical study of severely ill and therefore presumably highly compliant patients no further evidence of compliance was collected otherwise than the signature of the nurse on the medication chart. Fifteen patients were removed from the trial, three because of sudden cardiac death, two because of heart attack, and ten because of need for more intensive therapy (four underwent emergency percutaneous transluminal coronary angioplasty (PTCA) or coronary artery bypass graphting because of more than 70% left anterior descending (LAD) proximal stenoses or three-vessel disease). Of the dropouts 7 were in the celiprolol, 8 were in the propranolol group. Of the remaining 53 patients 13 were scheduled for elective surgery or PTCA. In the meantime they completed the trial, as did the other patients who were not scheduled for surgery. There were no asymmetries in the patients' characteristics (Table I). Many had elevated 24 hour excretions of metanephrines, indicating that their cardiac condition produced a significant increase of neurohumoral sympathetic activity. The pre-study time frames were balanced and similar in the two treatment groups both for admission with crescendo angina to attempted mobilisation (generally 24 hours) and attempted mobilisation to recording of baseline data (except for the weekends in most patients coronary angiography was performed the same day; so, they could be scheduled for the trial within the next 24 hours). All patients

TABLE I

Patients' characteristics.

	Celiprolol n = 26	p	Propranolol n = 27
Mean age (range)	67.7 years (40–81)	n.s.	64.0 years (36–84)
Males/females	16/10	n.s.	14/13
Mean number of coronary arteries stenosed by > 50% (S.D.)	1.8 (1.0)	n.s.	1.7 (0.8)
Smoking	34%	n.s.	30%
Mean weight (range)	82.2 kg (65–102)	n.s.	84.1 kg (48–90)
Mean cholesterol (S.D.)	7.3 mmol/l (2.4)	n.s.	7.5 mmol/l (2.1)
Mean blood pressure (S.D.)	150/82 mm Hg (12/9)	n.s.	148/80 mm Hg (12/9)
Mean 24-hour excretion of metanephrines (range)*	3.8 mmol/24 hours (1.8–5.9)	n.s.	3.9 mmol/24 hours (1.9–12.0)

* Reference range 0.006–3.8 mmol/24 hours.

were enrolled in a regimen of blood pressure, heart rate, and fore-arm blood flow measurements every 1–2 hours for 7 days. Forearm blood flow was measured by iridium strain gauge venous occlusion plethysmography. In addition, supine blood pressure, heart rate, fore-arm blood flow, and a 12-lead electrocardiogram were recorded during anginal attacks prior to the administration of sublingual nitroglycerin. An anginal attack was defined as typical pain in combination with more than 1 mm ST-segment depression in at least one of the leads of a 12-lead electrocardiogram. ST-segment depression was not taken into account when occurring without pain or on the monitor strip only. Also a diary of number of anginal attacks was kept both by patient and nurse. Of the 53 patients a subgroup of 25 (12 on celiprolol, 13 on propranolol) was studied for left ventricular function (in the absence of angina pectoris), at entry, and after 7 days' treatment. For estimation of left ventricular function supine ejection fraction and cardiac output were measured by use of serial M Mode echocardiograms with a 5" megahertz transducer according to Teichholz [12].

STATISTICS

Univariate within- and between-subject analyses were performed by use of student's t-tests for continuous and chi-square tests for binary data. In addition, Wilcoxon's tests were performed for the daily rates of anginal attacks, because these data were not normally distributed. We performed a stepwise logistic regression analysis [13] of the determinants of persistent angina in order to determine dependent and independent variables. For that purpose patients were divided into two new groups. They were assigned to the "no angina group" if they had 0–1 anginal attacks daily after 1 week irrespective of the type of treatment, to the "persistent angina group" if they had two or more anginal attacks daily. We entered all the variables of the univariate analysis except for the left ventricular function variables that were not included because of incomplete data and little effect of these variables in the univariate analysis. After adjusting for the independent variables we calculated the odds ratio (OR) of persistent angina pectoris in the celiprolol and the propranolol group.

$$OR = \frac{\text{incidence persistent angina pectoris in the celiprolol group}}{\text{incidence persistent angina pectoris in the propranolol group}}$$

7.3. Results

Table II shows the effects of 1 week treatment with either celiprolol or propranolol on the hemodynamic variables and the clinical symptoms versus baseline. Nearly all patients had angina pectoris stage IV NYHA at baseline, in addition to important ST-segment depressions and they all consumed large amounts of nitroglycerin tablets. After 1 week angina pectoris stage III–IV had become stage 0–I in both the celiprolol and the propranolol group. However, angina frequency was significantly higher in the propranolol group than in the celiprolol group. So were mean ST-segment depression and nitroglycerin consumption although the latter was not significant. For the estimation of the hemodynamic differences we took the values during the anginal attacks or took highest values of the day. Systolic blood pressure fell somewhat on celiprolol, it increased on propranolol. The same thing happened to diastolic blood pressure, though not significantly. Heart rate slightly fell

TABLE II

Comparison of changes from baseline for celiprolol and propranolol treatment groups (mean ± SD)°.

		Celiprolol n = 26	p	Propranolol n = 27
Systolic blood	1	148±12	n.s.	145±12
pressure (mm Hg)	2	136±12**	< 0.001	155±12**
Diastolic blood	1	81±9	n.s.	81±9
pressure (mm Hg)	2	78±9	n.s.	83±9
Heart rate	1	78±9	n.s.	76±9
(beats/min)	2	70±8**	< 0.01	64±8**
Double-product	1	111±11	n.s.	111±11
(beats/min.mm Hg × 10^2)	2	96±10***	n.s.	100±10**
Forearm blood flow	1	5.2±2.1	n.s.	5.6±2.4
(ml/100 ml tissue.min)	2	8.7±2.4**	< 0.001	3.7±1.9*
Angina pectoris	1	6 (3–16)	n.s.	6 (4–20)
(daily attack rate)	2	1 (0–4)***	< 0.01	2 (0–9)**
ST-segment depression	1	4.3±2.1**	n.s.	4.1±2.1
(mm)	2	1.2±1.1	< 0.01	2.3±1.5*
Daily number of nitro-				
glycerin Tab's	1	7.5±2.7	n.s.	6.4±2.5
required	2	1.9±1.4**	n.s.	2.1±1.5***
Left ventricular	1	55±7	n.s.	55±7
ejection fraction (%)	2	52±7	n.s.	53±7
n = 12 v n = 13				
Cardiac output	1	5.2±1.7	n.s.	5.6±1.7
(liter/min)	2	5.8±2.4	< 0.05	4.5±1.7*
n = 12 v n = 13				
Stroke volume	1	67±10	n.s.	73±11
(ml)	2	82±11*	< 0.05	70±10

° Angina pectoris rating was expressed as medians and range because these values were somewhat skewed to the right.
[1] baseline.
[2] 1 week treatment.
* $p < 0.05$ versus baseline.
** $p < 0.01$ versus baseline.
*** $p < 0.001$ versus baseline.

on celiprolol. This effect was much more pronounced on propranolol. The increase of systolic blood pressure on propranolol and the large reduction of heart rate still resulted in a reduction of the double-product on propranolol which was similar to celiprolol. The effects on forearm blood flow of the two compounds were largely different. Propranolol significantly reduced flow, while celiprolol largely increased flow. The effects on left ventricular function of the two compounds were small. Ejection fractions were not influenced. Although propranolol reduced cardiac output somewhat, the effect was exclusively due to a reduction of the heart rate and not to a change of the stroke volume. Table III shows the results after 1 week beta-blocker treatment, when patients were divided into two new groups, irrespective of the type of beta-blocker they had had. Systolic blood pressure was significantly higher in the persistent angina group. So were diastolic blood pressure and heart rate, though less significantly. The double-product was essentially higher in the persistent angina pectoris group while forearm blood flow was lower. Also treatment with propranolol was significantly more frequent in the persistent angina pectoris group compared to the group with few complaints. In the logistic regression analysis the variables from Table III were entered. We determined that the double-product and the treatment assignment were the only independent variables ($p < 0.0005$ and $p < 0.002$). After removal of the double-product as a variable, heart rate, treatment assignment and systolic blood pressure were the only independent variables ($p < 0.001$, $p < 0.002$ and $p < 0.005$). The remaining variables including flow, although largely different in the univariate analysis were not significant anymore. This indicates that flow is not independent but is largely dependent on treatment assignment. After adjustment for treatment assignment the difference in flow is no more significant. Also, after removal of the double-product from the variables, the difference in flow is no more significant. These results support that celiprolol acts beneficially through its vasodilatory property. This is furthermore supported by the odds ratios of persistent angina (Table IV). In our material celiprolol is capable of controlling unstable angina in three times as many patients as propranolol. After adjustment for the independent variables it does so even in eight times as many patients. Apparently, when the benefit of the double-product is removed by the adjustment, no further benefit of propranolol is left in

TABLE III

Angina pectoris after 1 week (mean ± SD).

	No angina pectoris n = 23	p	Persistent angina pectoris n = 30
Systolic blood pressure (mm Hg)	134±17	< 0.001	155±19
Diastolic blood pressure (mm Hg)	77±13	< 0.02	84±9
Heart rate (beats/min)	65±9	< 0.09	69±9
Double-product (beats/min.mm Hg × 10^2)	86±11	< 0.0001	107±14
Forearm blood flow (ml/100 ml tissue.min)	8.8±10.8	< 0.02	4.1±2.2
Treatment assignment (celiprolol/propranolol)	18/5	< 0.001	8/22

TABLE IV

Odds ratio of persistent angina in the celiprolol and propranolol group adjusted for the independent variables.

	Odds ratio	95% Confidence intervals	p Values
Unadjusted	0.38	0.25–0.52	< 0.002
Adjusted for double-product	0.13	0.05–0.22	< 0.0005
Adjusted for systolic blood pressure plus heart rate	0.12	0.04–0.20	< 0.0005

the data. Celiprolol, however, then starts performing even better probably because of its vasodilatory property which propranolol lacks.

7.4. Discussion

There are some weaknesses in our assessment. First, the use of fixed doses instead of a dose-ranging design might have provided a less adequate beta-blockade in some of our patients. However, we thought that 1 week treatment would be too short for reliably performing a more complex design. Also, a cardioselective beta-blocker instead of the nonselective beta-blocker propranolol is preferred by some cardiologists. However, there is no evidence in the literature so far that propranolol is actually less effective. Secondly, we chose a selected subset of patients to address a particular physiologic issue. This means that our results can only be applied to those patients with persistent signs or symptoms following bed rest and other standard medical therapies. In addition, in some practices beta-blockers are used only in patients with increased heart rates rather than routinely. The conclusions from our study are therefore of a preliminary nature and will have to be confirmed by others as well as tested in a broader perspective.

Celiprolol is a beta-1-selective beta-blocker and lacks, thus, beta-2-receptor blocking capacity. This may be advantageous in ischemic heart disease because beta-2-receptor blockade has been associated with peripheral vasoconstriction giving rise to increase of afterload. In addition, it exerts a direct vasodilatory activity, presumably by a beta-2-selective agonistic property which may have additional advantage in ischemic heart disease because of afterload reduction. In spite of these theoretically beneficial properties, celiprolol has not been proven to be unequivocally more efficient than other beta-blockers. Previous studies [10, 14–19], however, have focused on exercise-induced angina pectoris and not on unstable angina pectoris at rest. To test the afterload reduction hypothesis exercise-induced angina pectoris is probably not an appropriate model because local metabolic factors override the antagonistic effect on vasodilation during physical exercise. For example, Silke [15] found a difference of peripheral resistance between celiprolol and propranolol of more than 35% at rest, and of less than 15% during excercise. Prida [20] found no difference of peripheral resistance or benefit between selective and nonselective beta-blockers in exercise-induced angina pectoris. Apparently, exercise itself has an afterload reducing effect which interacts with the afterload reducing effect of the beta-blockers. This explains why differences between celiprolol and other beta-blockers are less impressive in the exercise studies than they are in our "at rest" study.

Nonetheless the trends given by the other studies are in agreement with our data. McLenachan et al. [18] and Frishman et al. [10] found a higher double-product at a given degree of exercise by celiprolol compared with either atenolol or propranolol. They attributed this beneficial effect on the myocardial oxygen balance to either afterload reduction or a positive inotropic effect. In our study equipotent doses of celiprolol and propranolol reduced the double-product similarly. However, angina frequency and ST depression were less severe on celiprolol. With similar levels of angina frequency and ST depression the double-product on celiprolol would probably have been essentially higher. So, actually, our data do confirm the results from the exercise studies. McLenachan [18] contended that measurement of left ventricular function variables can not prove whether the beneficial effect of celiprolol on myocardial oxygen balance compared to other beta-blockers is due to afterload reduction or a positive inotropic effect. This is true. However, the ratio of mean arterial pressure and cardiac output equals peripheral resistance, which can be used as estimate for afterload. Doing so Silke [15] found indeed that peripheral resistance on celiprolol was essentially lower than on atenolol in the absence of an increased cardiac output. These data are in agreement with our univariate data and support the belief that afterload reduction is a major mechanism in the beneficial effect of celiprolol. It is furthermore supported by our multivariate analysis showing the dependency of peripheral flow on the angina variables. On the other hand it is not easy to prove to what extent the general decrease of cardiac output by beta-blockers other than celiprolol [21, 22] is due either to a negative inotropic/chronotropic effect or to increased afterload. The decrease of cardiac output on propranolol by 20% in our material accompanied by a decrease of peripheral flow of more than 50% suggests that the former mechanism is secondary to the latter.

In conclusion, celiprolol and propranolol largely reduce angina pectoris frequency and patients with unstable angina pectoris. In our material celiprolol is capable of controlling unstable angina in three times as many patients as propranolol. After adjustment for the change in systolic blood pressure times heart rate, it does so even in eight times as many patients. The similar effects of the two compounds on the double-product and the significantly different effect on peripheral blood flow support the theory that celiprolol exerts its beneficial effect through its vasodilatory property, in addition to reduction of the double-product.

Acknowledgements

I am indebted to Westminster Publications INC., New York, NY, and Mosby-Year Book INC, Philadelphia, PA, for kindly granting permission to use parts of papers previously published in ANGIOLOGY (1995; 46: 131–138), and Clin Pharmacol Ther (1995; 57: 50–56) respectively.

References

1. Beta-blocker heart attack trial research group: A randomized trial of propranolol in patients with acute myocardial infarction. JAMA 247: 1107–1114, 1982.
2. Miami trial research group: Metoprolol in acute myocardial infarction, a randomized placebo-controlled international study. Eur Heart J 6: 199–214, 1985.
3. Isis-1 group: Randomized trial of intravenous atenolol among 16,027 cases of suspected myocardial infarction. Lancet ii: 57–66, 1986.
4. Hoffman BB, Lefkowitz RJ: Adrenergic receptor antagonists. In: The pharmacological basis of therapeutics. Goodman and Gilman, New York: Pergamon Press, p 232, 1991.
5. Cleophas TJ, Kauw FH: Pressor responses from noncardioselective beta-blockers. Angiology 39: 587–596, 1988.
6. Cleophas TJ, Stapper GJ: A pressor effect of noncardioselective beta-blockers in mildly hypertensive during acute hospitalization. Angiology 41: 124–132, 1990.
7. Cleophas TJ, v. Asselt LM, Oudshoorn NH, Quadir SJ: A pressor effect of noncardioselective beta-blockers in mildly hypertensive patients during surgery under anesthesia. Angiology 42: 805–811, 1991.
8. Selwyn AP, Braunwald E.: Ischemic heart disease. In: Harrison's principles of internal medicine. Wilson JD, et al., New York: McGraw-Hill Inc, pp 964–971, 1991.
9. Fogari R, Zoppi A, Pasotti C: Plasma lipids during chronic antihypertensive therapy with different beta-blockers. J Cardiovasc Pharmacol 14 (suppl 7): 28–32, 1989.
10. Frishman WH, Heiman M, Soberman J, Greenberg S, Ett J, for the Celiprolol International Angina Study Group: Comparison of celiprolol and propranolol in stable angina pectoris. Am J Cardiol 67: 665–670, 1991.
11. Taylor SH, Beattie A, Silke B: Celiprolol in the treatment of hypertension: a comparison with propranolol. J Cardiovasc Pharmacol 8 (suppl): 127–131, 1986.
12. Teichholz LE: Problems in echocardiographic volume determinations: echocardiographic-angiographic correlations in the presence of asynergy. Am J Cardiol 37: 7–11, 1976.
13. SPSS Statistical Software, SPSS Inc, Chicago, 1988.

CHAPTER 7

14. Opie L: Qualities of an ideal beta-adrenoceptor antagonist and comparison of existing agents with a new cardioselective hydrophilic vasodilator beta-adrenoceptor antagonist, celiprolol. Am J Cardiol 61: 8–13, 1988.
15. Silke B, Verma SP, Frais MA, Reynolds G, Taylor SH: Differential actions of atenolol and celiprolol on cardiac performance in ischemic heart disease. J Cardiovasc Pharmacol 8 (suppl 4): 138–144, 1986.
16. Douard H, Koch M, Laporte T, Abella ML, Provendier V, Broustet JP: Anti-ischemic effects of celiprolol in patients with exercise-induced angina pectoris. Int J Cardiol 25: 63–68, 1989.
17. McLenachan J, Findlay JN, Henderson E, Wilson JT, Dargie AJ: Atenolol and celiprolol for stable angina pectoris (abstract). Am J Cardiol 61: 52, 1988.
18. McLenachan J, Wilson J, Dargie H: Improved left ventricular function during exercise: a comparison of celiprolol and atenolol. Am Heart J 1435–1436, 1988.
19. Soberman JE, Frishman WH: Celiprolol in angina pectoris. Am Heart J 116: 1422–1425, 1988.
20. Prida XE, Feldman RL, Hill JA, Pepine CJ: Comparison of selective and nonselective beta-adrenergic blockade on systemic and coronary hemodynamic findings in angina pectoris. Am J Cardiol 60: 244–248, 1987.
21. Solomon T, Gensini G, Dator C, Caruso F: Celiprolol: a haemodynamic appraisal in comparison with propranolol. Br J Clin Pract 39 (suppl): 43–44, 1985.
22. Mancia G: The central and peripheral hemodynamics of celiprolol. Am Heart J 116: 1405–1411, 1988.

CHAPTER 8

MORE ON PARADOXICAL PRESSOR EFFECTS OF NONSELECTIVE BETA-BLOCKERS

Background. Pressor effects have been described with nonselective beta-blockers, especially in situations of increased sympathetic activity.

Methods and Results. We give a review of the published data on this subject. Patients with high baseline plasma levels of epinephrine seem to be especially at risk; e.g., patients with unstable diabetes type I, sportsmen who perform a lot of isometric exercise, and perhaps also heavy smokers. The pressor effect is a reproducible phenomenon in patients with unstable angina pectoris, surgery, acute psychosis, and acute hospitalization.

Conclusions. Although the clinical relevance of the phenomenon in terms of permanent harm has not been elucidated so far, we may ask: do we require the very proof of it by exposing mankind to a less effective, and potentially hazardous compound.

8.1. The First Reports

A pressor effect of nonselective beta-blockers has been reported from the very beginning [1]. It was observed in patients with emotional stress, low renin hypertension and increased sympathetic activity [2], also in patients with untreated pheochromocytoma [3], with clonidine withdrawal [4], abuse of cocaine [5], and subcutaneous administration of epinephrine [6]. The most consistent finding in these reports was the situation of increased sympathetic activity. It was hypothesized that alpha-receptor-mediated vasoconstriction unopposed by beta-2-receptor-mediated vasodilation might be responsible. In situations of increased sympathetic activity this mechanism might override the otherwise hypotensive activity of nonselective beta-blockers. In order to test this hypothesis investigators started to design controlled trials comparing beta-1-selective and nonselective beta-blockers. On the one hand beta-1-selective blockers have a weak binding potency at the beta-2-receptor site and are, thus, less likely to produce this pressor effect. On the other hand, however, the selectivity is not absolute, but dose-dependent (e.g., metoprolol and atenolol lose their beta-1-selectivity with incremental doses [7]). Correspondingly, the different effects of beta-1-selective drugs on peripheral vascular resistance compared to nonselective compounds seem to be dose dependent [8]. Finally, even the heart does contain not only socalled cardioselective beta-1- but also otherwise vasodilative beta-2-adrenergic receptors [9].

8.2. Controlled Studies Designed to Demonstrate Pressor Responses from Nonselective Beta-Blockers

INFUSIONS OF EPINEPHRINE

If epinephrine is administered mean arterial pressure hardly changes. This is so because epinephrine stimulates both alpha- and beta-receptors. Alpha-receptor stimulation causes vasoconstriction, beta-2-receptor stimulation vasodilation. The net effect is that mean arterial pressure remains essentially unchanged. The effect is different if patients have been pretreated with a nonselective beta-blocker. Pretreatment with propranolol, e.g., causes an increase of mean arterial pressure of 20–30 mm Hg, because the vasodilative beta-2-receptors are blocked by nonselective beta-blockers, and, thus, epinephrine is no longer capable of a vasodilative effect. This very thing does not happen in case of pretreatment with, e.g., metoprolol or atenolol, beta-1-selective blockers, because of their low binding potency at the beta-2-receptor site. By now this phenomenon has been reported by four groups, so it can not be easily ignored [10]. The effect has not yet been examined in patients with enhanced receptor sensitivity: patients with acute anxiety syndromes overreact to infusion of epinephrine compared to psychologically stable subjects [11]. Neither has the effect been examined after administration of norepinephrine which is a more potent vasoconstrictor than epinephrine. This is even more important because 2 kinds of sympathetic overactivity have been recognized: a norepinephrine-effect by release of norepinephrine from the sympathetic nerve endings, and a epinephrine-effect mainly mediated by indirect release of epinephrine from the adrenal medulla [12], nowadays also called the aggressive and defensive sympathetic reaction respectively. Moreover, there are miscellaneous forms (like, e.g., handgrip). Obviously, daily life stress involves more complicated processes than the infusion of epinephrine does.

PHARMACOLOGIC STRESS

In normotensive subjects who are being treated with saline or atenolol blood pressure is hardly influenced by two cigarettes [22]. Pretreatment with propranolol, however, does cause a significant rise of diastolic blood pressure of 12 mm Hg. The same effect is seen after chronic treatment with nonselective beta-blockers, as reported by three groups [10]. Nicotine is – just like caffeine and insulin – a drug in daily life that causes a substantial rise of plasma epinephrine and can, thus, be used as a model for pharmacologic stress [10]. As a matter of fact, insulin has been quite successful in demonstrating a pressor response from propranolol [10] (increase of diastolic blood pressure from 80 to 90 mm Hg), whereas pretreatment with beta-1-selective beta-blockers even caused a slight decrease of diastolic blood pressure from 80 to 65 mm Hg. What about caffeine ? It has been less successful than nicotine and insulin. In some studies no difference was found between pretreatment with a beta-1-selective and a nonselective beta-blocker [10]. This failure was ascribed to an increase of plasma epinephrine of less than 200%, which was the lowest level to cause a pressor response to infusion of epinephrine. Much more coffee would be needed or the same quantity together with a bit of nicotine as demonstrated by Freestone [13]. After pretreatment with the nonselective beta-blocker oxprenolol for 6 weeks, 500 ml coffee and 2 cigarettes caused an increase of systolic blood pressure of 12.1 ± 3.6 mm Hg and of the diastolic blood pressure of 9.1 ± 2.6 mm Hg (both $p < 0.01$). Other workers, however, did find that the pressor effect disappeared in heavy smokers after more than 4 week treatment [14]. What little is absolutely true is documented by the paper of Shepherd [15] reporting an increase from 140/80 to 230/112 mm Hg during hypoglycaemia in a patient who had been treated with the beta-1-selective blocker metoprolol for many years. Finally, whether the absence of any cardiovascular response to hypoglycaemia is a true advantage, is uncertain.

OTHER TYPES OF STRESS

Other types of stress to study differences between the two beta-blockers are 1. environmental stress, such as cold, loud noise, pain; 2. mental stress, such as arithmetic; 3. physical stress, e.g., handgrip and different types of dynamic exercise. Most of these stress models cause smaller increases of catecholamines in the laboratory than the infusion of catecholamines does [10]. Nonetheless, subtle differences between beta-1-selective and nonselective beta-blockers could repeatedly be demonstrated. E.g., loud noise caused a significant increase of blood pressure of 10 mm Hg and also of peripheral vascular resistance in hypertensive patients treated with propranolol [10]. In the case of metoprolol this was not so. Similar effects of nonselective beta-blockers were observed with mental arithmetic and physical stress tests such as handgrip. The effects were demonstrated both in acute and chronic studies [10]. After dynamic exercise, local metabolic factors probably override the antagonistic effect on vasodilation. However, in a category of low anaerobic metabolism, namely long-distance runners, performance was impaired by 30% when the subjects received propranolol but by only 10% when they received atenolol. Karlson [16] attributed this effect to prevention of beta-2-receptor-mediated vasodilation. In recent years controlled and double-blind studies on pressor effects of nonselective beta-blockers have been performed in patients with acute psychosis [17], acute hospitalization [18], surgery [19], unstable angina pectoris [20]. During surgery under anesthesia an increase of blood pressure is generally no problem. The anesthesiologist generally has less a problem with high than with low blood pressure because of the hypotensive effects of most anesthetic drugs. In unstable angina pectoris an increase of blood pressure of 30 mm Hg is certainly unfavorable because the double-product (systolic blood pressure × heart rate) which is an estimate of myocardial oxygen demand increases. Nonselective beta-blockers were as a matter of fact less effective than beta-1-selective beta-blockers in unstable angina pectoris [18, 20].

8.3. Other Studies Demonstrating Pressor Responses from Nonselective Beta-Blockers

ALPHA-BLOCKADE

As can be seen, the pressor responses appear exclusively in situations of increased sympathetic activity. An increased release of norepinephrine from sympathetic nerve terminals and increased levels of plasma norepinephrine are consistent findings in patients on nonselective alpha-blockers. This is so because blockade of alpha-2-receptors that are present on the sympathetic nerve endings enhances largely the release of norepinephrine. Consequently, this may be a situation to demonstrate a pressor response from nonselective beta-blockers as well. Indeed, in young hypertensive patients the nonselective alpha-blocker phentolamine caused a mean fall in blood pressure of 16.5 mm Hg and an increase in mean heart rate of 19 beats/min. After pretreatment with propranolol the mean fall in blood pressure was only 4.7 mm Hg (before versus after $p < 0.01$), whereas heart rate hardly increased [21]. Also other groups have demonstrated that propranolol antagonizes not only the increase in heart rate but also the hypotensive activity of nonselective alpha-blockers [10]. On the other hand, no such effect can be expected from the more modern alpha-1-selective alpha-blockers like prazosine that block predominantly the vasoconstrictive postsynaptic alpha-1-receptors. The absence of a protective effect against hypotension in another study [22], shows that it is a subtle mechanism we are dealing with: if a pressor effect due to beta-2-blockade is counteracted by a vasodilator effect via the alpha-receptors and a decrease of cardiac output via the beta-1-receptors the net effect may as well be a considerable decrease of blood pressure.

AUTONOMIC NEUROPATHY

Orthostatic hypotension based on autonomic neuropathy has been treated successfully with nonselective beta-blockers, although most reports were case histories without control observations [10]. To eliminate potential biases as seen with uncontrolled studies we performed a double-blind placebo-controlled study in 11 patients with symptoms of orthostatic hypotension [23]. All patients had vagal neuropathy and largely elevated levels of plasma catecholamines as seen with hyper-adrenergic diabetic syndrome. Different beta-agonists (terbutaline and orciprenaline) did not reduce the fall of blood pressure on standing. The beta-1-blockers acebutolol and metoprolol did neither. Only, the nonselective beta-blockers propranolol and pindolol significantly reduced or practically abolished the fall. This effect was confirmed by a three week trial with pindolol [23]. As cardiac output was reduced, the effect was ascribed, not to positive inotropic intrinsic sympathicomimetic activity effect, but rather to prevention of beta-2-receptor vasodilation. Roughly, orthostatic hypotension can be distributed in two categories, a hypoadrenergic with very low and a hyperadrenergic form with very high plasma catecholamine levels. The former category may benefit from intrinsic sympathicomimetic activity [24], and from beta-1-agonists like xamoterol [25]. The latter category probably does not, because beta-receptors are already stimulated maximally. This explains why xamoterol did not have any beneficial effect in diabetics with orthostatic hypotension and presumably hyperadrenergic status [26].

8.4. Conclusions

Paradoxical pressor effects of nonselective beta-blockers have been reported in more than 60 papers. The pressor effects are probably due to alpha-receptor-mediated vasoconstriction unopposed by beta-2-receptor-mediated vasodilation. In situations of increased sympathetic activity this mechanism may override the otherwise hypotensive properties of nonselective beta-blockers. Some patients seem to be at risk; e.g., patients with unstable diabetes type I, sportsmen who perform a lot of isometric exercise, heavy smokers. In them the preference for a beta-1-selective beta-blocker seems reasonable. In 1988 we reviewed the papers on this subject so far. Our conclusions have been adopted by Goodman and Gilman, "The pharmacological basis of therapeutics" [27]. In recent controlled and double blind studies the pressor effect has been demonstrated during increased sympathetic activity due to unstable angina pectoris [20], surgery [19], acute hospitalization [18]. Although the clinical relevance of the phenomenon in terms of permanent harm has not been elucidated so far, we may ask: do we require the very proof of it by exposing mankind to a less effective, and potentially hazardous compound. Beta-2-blockade, if not hazardous, does

TABLE I
Beta-1-selective and nonselective beta-blockers.

	Beta-1-selective	ISA*	Alpha-blockade
Acebutolol	+	+/-	–
Alprenolol	–	+	–
Atenolol	++	–	–
Betaxolol	++	–	–
Bevantolol	++	–	–
Bisoprolol	++	–	–
Carvedilol	–	–	+
Celiprolol	++	+	–
Esmolol	++	–	–
Labetalol	–	–	+
Metoprolol	++	–	–
Oxprenolol	–	++	–
Pindolol	–	+++	–
Propranolol	–	–	–
Sotalol	–	–	–
Tertatolol	–	–	–
Timolol	–	–	–

+, ++, +++ = extent to which effect is present.
– = effect is not present.
* ISA = intrinsic sympathicomimetic activity.

not help reducing blood pressure either [28], although initially it was thought to be so [29]. We should add that there are more reasons for choosing a beta-1-selective blocker, e.g., bronchus constriction especially in patients with chronic obstructive pulmonary disease, delayed recovery from hypoglycaemia in diabetes mellitus, and severe hypertriglyceridaemia. The pressor effects have also been described with nonselective beta-blockers with intrinsic sympathicomimetic activity (Table I) [30] or with additional alpha-blocker property (labetalol) [31]. This is not too much of a surprise because these compounds do block beta-2-receptors, although maybe less vigorously. Moreover, labetalol is not that good for additional alpha-1-blockade since it lacks alpha-1-selectivity. Carvedilol which is alpha-1-selective may be a better choice, but even this compound does block beta-2-receptors.

The reverse of the medal is that the results of secondary prevention studies of myocardial infarction are slightly in favor of nonselective beta-blockers. Maybe, this is partly due to the presence of mostly normotensives in this category. Still, even in these patients the beneficial effect of nonselective beta-blockade is lost by the factor smoking [32].

Acknowledgements

I am indebted to American Heart Association, Dallas, TX, for kindly granting permission to use part of a paper published in CIRCULATION (1994; 90: 2157–2158).

References

1. Prichard BNC: Hypotensive action of pronethalol. Br Med J 1: 1227–1228, 1964.
2. Drayer JIM, Keim HJ, Weber MA, Case DB, Laragh JH: Unexpected pressor response to propranolol in essential hypertension on interaction between renin, aldosterone, and sympathetic activity. Am J Med 60: 896–903, 1976.
3. Bravo El, Gifford RW: Pheochromocytoma: diagnosis, localization and management. N Engl J Med 311: 1298–1303, 1987.
4. Strauss FG, Franklin SS, Lewin AJ, Maxwell MH: Withdrawal of antihypertensive therapy. JAMA 238: 1734–1736, 1977.
5. Ramoska E, Sachetti AD: Propranolol-induced hypertension in treatment of cocaine-intoxication. Ann Emerg Med 14: 112–113, 1985.
6. Foster CA, Aston SJ: Propranolol-epinephrine interaction: a potential disaster. Plast Reconstr Surg 72: 74–78, 1983.
7. Lipworth BJ, Irvin NA, Mc Devitt DG: The effects of time and dose on the relative β_1- and β_2-adrenoceptor antagonism of betaxolol and atenolol. Br J Clin Pharmacol 31: 154–159, 1991.
8. Kelbaek H, Godtfredsen J: Effect of acute cardioselective and non-selective beta-adrenergic blockade on left-ventricular volumes and vascular resistance at rest and during exercise. Scand J Clin Lab Invest 51: 161–166, 1991.
9. Brodde OE, Karad K, Zerkowski HR, Rohm N, Reidemeister JC: Coexistence of β_1- and β_2-adrenoceptors in human right atrium. Circ Res 53: 752–758, 1983.
10. Cleophas AJM, Kauw FHW: Pressor responses from noncardioselective β-blockers. Angiology 39: 587–596, 1988.
11. Pitts FN, Allen RE: β-Adrenergic blockade in the treatment of anxiety. Mathew RJ, ed. The biology of anxiety, proceedings of the 14th Annual Symposium. Houston, TX: Texas Research Institute of Mental Sciences 134–161, 1980.
12. Goodall MC, Stone C: Adrenaline and noradrenaline producing tumours of the adrenal medulla and sympathetic nerves. Anal Surg 151: 391–398, 1960.

13. Freestone S, Ramsay LE: Effect of beta-blockade on the pressor response to coffee plus smoking in patients with mild hypertension. Drugs 25(s): 141–145, 1983.
14. Houben H, Thien Th, van 't Laar: Haemodynamic effects of cigarette smoking during chronic selective and non-selective beta-adrenoceptor blockade in patients with hypertension. Br J Clin Pharmacol 12: 67–72, 1981.
15. Shepherd AMM, Lin MS, Keeton TK: Hypoglycemia-induced hypertension in a diabetic patient on metoprolol. Ann Intern Med 94: 357–358, 1981.
16. Karlson J: Muscle fiber composition, short-term beta-1 and beta-2 blockade and endurance exercise performance in healthy young men. Drugs 25(s): 241–246, 1983.
17. Atsmon A, Blum I, Steinger M: Further studies with propranolol in psychotic patients: Relation to initial psychiatric state, urinary catecholamines, and 3-methoxy-4-hydroxyglycol excretion. Psychopharmacologia 27: 249–254, 1972.
18. Cleophas TJ, Stapper GJ: A pressor effect of noncardioselective beta-blockers in mildly hypertensive patients during acute hospitalization. Angiology 41: 124–132, 1990.
19. Cleophas TJ, v. Asselt L, Oudshoorn N, Quadir S: A pressor effect of noncardioselective beta-blockers in mildly hypertensive patients during surgery under anaesthesia. Angiology 42: 805–811, 1991.
20. van 't Leven M, Cleophas TJ, Kauw FH, Remmert HP, Kuijper A, Zwinderman K: Celiprolol versus propranolol in unstable angina pectoris. Clin Pharmacol Ther 57: 50–56, 1995.
21. Zahir M, Could L: Phentolamine and beta-adrenergic receptors. J Clin Pharmacol 11: 197–203, 1971.
22. Beilin LJ, Juel-Jansen BE: α- and β-adrenergic blockade in hypertension. Lancet i: 979–982, 1972.
23. Cleophas TJM, Kauw FHW, Bijl CH: Effects of beta-adrenergic receptor agonists and antagonists in diabetics with symptoms of postural hypotension: A double-blind placebo-controlled study. Angiology 37: 855–862, 1986.
24. Man in 't Veld, Schalekamp MADH: Pindolol acts as beta-adrenoceptor agonist in orthostatic hypotension: Therapeutic implications. Br Med J 282: 929–931, 1981.
25. Mehlsen J, Stadeager C, Trap-Jensen J: Differential effects of beta-adrenoceptor partial agonists in patients with postural hypotension. Eur J Clin Pharmacol 44: 7–11, 1993.
26. Leslie PJ, Thomson C, Clarke BF, Ewing DJ: A double-blind crossover study of oral xamoterol in postural hypotension due to diabetic autonomic neuropathy. Clin Auton Res 1: 119–123, 1991.
27. Hoffman BB, Lefkowitz RJ: Beta-adrenergic receptor antagonists. Goodman Gilman A, Rall TW, Nies AS, et al., eds. The pharmacological basis of therapeutics. New York, NY: Pergamon Press, pp 221–244, 1991.
28. Dahlöf B, Andren L, Svensson A, Hansson L: Antihypertensive mechanisms of beta-adrenoceptor antagonism: the role of β-2-blockade. J Hypertens 1 (s2): 112–115, 1983.
29. Langer SZ: Presynaptic receptors and their role in the regulation of transmitter release. Br J Pharmacol 60: 481–497, 1977.
30. Bjerle P, Jacobsson KA, Agert G: Paradoxical effect of pindolol. Br Med J 4: 284, 1975.
31. Crofton M, Gabriel R: Pressor response after intravenous labetalol. Br Med J 2: 737, 1977.
32. Fox K, Jonathan A, Williams H, Selwyn A: Interaction between cigarettes and propranolol in treatment of angina pectoris. Br Med J 281: 191–193, 1980.